CHAIR YOGA FOR SENIORS ABOVE 60

A beginner's guide to unlock your
Mobility and flexibility in 15 minutes
Daily (loose weight in 21 days)

Haseeb Ahmad

CONTENTS

CHAPTER 1: INTRODUCTION TO CHAIR YOGA FOR SENIORS

As the aging process unfolds, maintaining an active and healthy lifestyle becomes increasingly crucial for seniors. Chair yoga, a gentle and accessible form of yoga, emerges as an excellent option for individuals above 60, offering a gateway to enhanced mobility, flexibility, and overall well-being. This introduction provides an in-depth exploration of chair yoga, shedding light on its origins, benefits, and the foundational principles that make it an ideal practice for seniors.

Origins of Chair Yoga:

Chair yoga is a modern adaptation of traditional yoga practices, catering specifically to those who may face challenges with traditional floor-based poses. The roots of chair yoga can be traced back to the late 20th century when yoga teachers and healthcare professionals recognized the need for modified practices to accommodate individuals with limited mobility or physical constraints.

The Essence of Chair Yoga:

At its core, chair yoga combines the wisdom of traditional yoga with modifications that make the practice accessible to seniors. The use of a chair provides support and stability, allowing participants to experience the benefits of yoga without the need for complex floor poses. This modified approach focuses on adapting traditional asanas, pranayama (breath control), and meditation techniques to a seated or supported position.

Getting Started with Chair Yoga:

Embarking on a chair yoga journey involves minimal setup and can be done in the comfort of one's home. A sturdy chair with a straight back and no armrests is ideal. Participants should wear comfortable clothing, and having a yoga mat or non-slip surface under the chair ensures stability.

Conclusion:

The introduction to chair yoga for seniors sets the stage for a transformative journey toward improved health and well-being. By providing a gentle yet effective approach to yoga, this practice empowers seniors to embrace a daily routine that fosters flexibility, mobility, and a holistic sense of balance. As we delve deeper into the subsequent chapters, we will explore specific chair yoga poses, breathing exercises, and sequences designed to unlock the full potential of this accessible and enriching practice for seniors above 60.

CHAPTER 2: THE BENEFITS OF CHAIR YOGA FOR INDIVIDUALS ABOVE 60

Chair yoga stands as a beacon of holistic wellness for individuals above 60, offering a treasure trove of physical, mental, and emotional benefits tailored to the unique needs of seniors. In this detailed exploration, we delve into the myriad advantages that chair yoga brings to this demographic, emphasizing how this gentle practice contributes to overall health and well-being.

Physical Benefits:

- **Improved Flexibility:** Chair yoga gently encourages a wide range of motion, promoting flexibility without putting undue stress on joints. Seniors can enjoy increased suppleness in muscles and joints, enhancing overall mobility.

- **Enhanced Joint Health:** The controlled and mindful movements in chair yoga contribute to the lubrication of joints, reducing stiffness and discomfort commonly associated with aging. This is particularly beneficial for individuals with conditions like arthritis.

- **Strengthening Muscles:** Seated poses engage various muscle groups, promoting strength and stability. This is crucial for maintaining functional independence and preventing muscle atrophy.

- **Better Circulation:** The rhythmic nature of chair yoga sequences, combined with focused breathing, supports healthy blood flow. Improved circulation can have positive effects on cardiovascular health and overall vitality.

- **Posture Improvement:** Chair yoga emphasizes awareness of body alignment and encourages proper posture. This focus on mindful positioning can help alleviate back pain and prevent issues related to poor posture.

Mental and Emotional Benefits:

- **Stress Reduction:** Chair yoga incorporates mindfulness and breath control, fostering a calming effect on the nervous system. Seniors can experience reduced stress levels, leading to improved overall mental well-being.

- **Enhanced Cognitive Function:** The combination of movement and mindfulness in chair yoga has been linked to improved cognitive function. Regular practice may contribute to better concentration, memory, and mental clarity.

- **Mood Elevation:** The release of endorphins during chair yoga can contribute to an uplifted mood. This is particularly significant for seniors who may face challenges such as isolation or depression.

- **Better Sleep:** Chair yoga's relaxation techniques can aid in promoting better sleep patterns. Seniors may find relief from insomnia or sleep disturbances through the calming effects of the practice.

Emotional Resilience and Mindfulness:

- **Coping with Aging Challenges:** Chair yoga provides a space for individuals to explore and accept the changes that come with aging. Mindfulness practices within chair yoga can foster emotional resilience, helping seniors navigate life's challenges with a positive mindset.

- **Building Mind-Body Connection:** The mindful nature of chair yoga encourages individuals to connect with their bodies. This mind-body awareness can deepen one's understanding of their physical and emotional states.

Social and Community Aspects:

- **Fostering Social Connections:** Group chair yoga classes can provide a sense of community and social interaction, combating feelings of loneliness or isolation that seniors may experience.

- **Accessible to All Fitness Levels:** Chair yoga is inclusive and can be adapted to various fitness levels, making it accessible to a wide range of individuals. This inclusivity fosters a sense of belonging for participants.

Long-Term Wellness and Independence:

- **Preventing Falls:** Improved balance and stability from chair yoga contribute to fall prevention, a crucial consideration for senior health and independence.

- **Empowering Self-Care:** Chair yoga empowers individuals to take an active role in their health. The daily practice of simple, yet effective, routines can instill a sense of agency and self-care.

Integrating Chair Yoga into Daily Life:

- **Creating a Routine:** The benefits of chair yoga compound with regular practice. Establishing a daily routine, even if it's just 15 minutes, can lead to sustained improvements in physical and mental well-being.

- **Adapting to Individual Needs:** Chair yoga can be tailored to individual abilities and needs, making it an adaptable practice for seniors with varying health conditions.

Conclusion:

In conclusion, the benefits of chair yoga for individuals above 60 extend far beyond the physical realm. This gentle practice emerges as a holistic approach to aging, addressing not only the body's changing needs but also nurturing mental resilience, emotional well-being, and social connections. As seniors embrace chair yoga, they embark on a journey of self-discovery and empowerment, unlocking a path to a more vibrant, balanced, and fulfilling life.

CHAPTER 3: SETTING UP YOUR SPACE FOR A SAFE AND COMFORTABLE PRACTICE

Creating an environment conducive to a safe and comfortable chair yoga practice is essential for individuals above 60. This detailed exploration focuses on the key elements of setting up a dedicated space, considering physical safety, comfort, and the overall ambience that enhances the chair yoga experience.

Physical Safety Considerations:

- **Choose the Right Chair:**
    - Ensure the chair used is sturdy, with a flat seat and a straight back.
    - Avoid chairs with wheels or armrests to prevent instability during poses.

- **Secure the Space:**
    - Clear the practice area of any potential hazards, such as loose rugs or clutter.
    - If practicing near furniture, make sure there's ample space to move without obstacles.

- **Non-Slip Surface:**
    - Place a non-slip mat or rug under the chair to prevent sliding, especially if practicing on hardwood or tile floors.

- **Proper Lighting:**
    - Ensure the practice space is well-lit to reduce the risk of tripping or missteps.

Creating a Comfortable Atmosphere:

- **Temperature Control:**

- Maintain a comfortable room temperature. Layers of clothing can be added or removed based on personal comfort.

- **Ventilation:**
  - Ensure good airflow in the room to prevent overheating during the practice.

- **Comfortable Clothing:**
  - Wear loose, comfortable clothing that allows for unrestricted movement.

- **Cushioning:**
  - Use cushions or pillows for additional support, especially if the chair is firm or if additional elevation is needed for certain poses.

- **Personalizing the Space:**
  - Decorate the space with items that bring joy and a sense of calm, such as plants, candles, or soothing colors.

Setting Up Technological Components:

- **Device Placement:**
  - If following an online chair yoga class, ensure the device (phone, tablet, or computer) is positioned at eye level to avoid straining the neck.

- **Internet Connection:**
  - Ensure a stable internet connection if streaming classes online to minimize disruptions during the practice.

Organizing Props and Accessories:

- **Yoga Props:**
  - Have any necessary props, such as blocks or resistance bands, within easy reach for added support during certain poses.

- **Water and Towel:**
  - Keep a water bottle nearby to stay hydrated and have a towel on hand for any perspiration.

Mindful Arrangement of the Space:

- **Dedicated Area:**
  - Designate a specific area for chair yoga practice to create a sense of ritual and focus.

- **Visual Appeal:**
  - Arrange the space with aesthetics in mind, incorporating elements that inspire a positive and calming atmosphere.

Preparation for Variations in Practice:

- **Adaptable Layout:**
  - Ensure the space is versatile to accommodate different chair yoga sequences and modifications.

- **Storage Solutions:**
  - Have a designated space to store yoga props and accessories when not in use to maintain an organized practice area.

Cultivating a Mindful Environment:

- **Silence or Soothing Sounds:**
  - Opt for a quiet environment or play soft, calming music to enhance the meditative aspects of chair yoga.

- **Distraction-Free Zone:**
  - Minimize external distractions by turning off phones or choosing a time when the household is relatively quiet.

Personalizing the Experience:

- **Aromatherapy:**
  - Consider incorporating aromatherapy through

essential oils or scented candles for an added sensory dimension.

- **Personal Affirmations:**
    - Create a positive space by incorporating personal affirmations or quotes that inspire and motivate.

Conclusion:

In conclusion, setting up a space for chair yoga is a multi-faceted endeavor that combines considerations for physical safety, comfort, and the creation of a mindful environment. By paying attention to these details, individuals above 60 can establish a dedicated and inviting space that supports a safe, comfortable, and transformative chair yoga practice, enhancing both physical and mental well-being.

CHAPTER 4: ESSENTIAL WARM-UP AND STRETCHING EXERCISES

Embarking on a chair yoga journey for individuals above 60 necessitates a thoughtful and comprehensive warm-up routine. This detailed exploration focuses on the importance of warming up the body, providing an array of essential chair yoga warm-up and stretching exercises. These preparatory activities not only enhance flexibility but also ensure a safe and enjoyable practice, promoting overall well-being.

Importance of Warm-up:

Before delving into specific exercises, it's crucial to understand the significance of a proper warm-up. A warm-up serves several key purposes:

- **Increased Blood Flow:** Gentle movements increase blood circulation, delivering oxygen and nutrients to muscles and joints.

- **Improved Flexibility:** Warm muscles and joints are more pliable, making it easier to engage in stretches and poses.

- **Joint Lubrication:** Movement during a warm-up aids in the production of synovial fluid, lubricating joints for smoother motion.

- **Injury Prevention:** Gradual warm-up reduces the risk of strains, sprains, and other injuries by preparing the body for physical activity.

Chair Yoga Warm-up Routine:

1. Seated Neck Stretches:

- Gently tilt the head to one side, holding for 10-15 seconds, and then switch to the other side.
- Slowly roll the neck in clockwise and counterclockwise motions to release tension.

2. **Shoulder Rolls:**

- Lift the shoulders toward the ears, roll them backward, and then downward in a circular motion.
- Repeat this for 10-15 seconds, then reverse the direction.

3. **Wrist and Ankle Circles:**

- Rotate the wrists and ankles in circular motions to improve mobility and flexibility in these joints.

4. **Seated Spinal Twist:**

- Sit with a straight back, twist the torso to one side, holding onto the chair for support.
- Hold for 15-20 seconds, then switch to the other side.

5. **Seated Forward Bend:**

- Sit at the edge of the chair, feet flat on the ground. Hinge at the hips, reaching toward the toes.
- Hold the stretch for 15-20 seconds, feeling a gentle stretch in the hamstrings and lower back.

6. **Knee Lifts:**

- Lift one knee toward the chest, holding onto the chair for balance. Hold for 10 seconds.
- Lower the leg and switch to the other side. This warms up the hip flexors and thighs.

7. **Ankle Flex and Point:**

- Lift one foot off the ground and flex the ankle, then point the toes.
- Repeat for 10-15 seconds and switch to the other foot.

8. **Seated Cat-Cow Stretch:**

  - Sit tall in the chair, arch the back and look up (Cow), then round the back and tuck the chin (Cat).
  - Flow between these movements for 1-2 minutes to warm up the spine.

9. **Seated Marching:**

  - Lift one knee at a time in a marching motion while seated to engage the core and warm up the hips.

10. **Deep Breathing:**

  - Finish the warm-up with deep, slow breaths. Inhale through the nose, expanding the belly, and exhale through the mouth, releasing tension.

Guidelines for an Effective Warm-up:

  - **Gradual Progression:** Ease into each movement, gradually increasing the range of motion.
  - **Pain-Free Range:** Avoid any exercise that causes pain. Discomfort is normal, but sharp pain should be avoided.
  - **Breath Awareness:** Coordinate breath with movement to enhance relaxation and focus.
  - **Individual Adaptations:** Modify exercises based on individual comfort and ability levels.

Conclusion:

In conclusion, the essential warm-up and stretching exercises for chair yoga are a foundational component of a safe and enjoyable practice for individuals above 60. This routine not only prepares the body for the subsequent yoga session but also contributes to improved flexibility, joint health, and overall well-being. By incorporating these gentle movements into a daily routine, individuals can unlock the full benefits of chair yoga, promoting physical and mental vitality in their journey towards enhanced health and mobility.

CHAPTER 5: CHAIR YOGA POSES FOR IMPROVED POSTURE

Posture plays a pivotal role in the overall well-being of individuals, particularly as they age. For seniors above 60, maintaining good posture becomes essential for preventing discomfort, reducing the risk of injuries, and promoting a positive self-image. This detailed exploration focuses on chair yoga poses specifically designed to enhance posture, providing a comprehensive guide to the benefits, techniques, and variations that contribute to improved spinal alignment and overall body awareness.

Importance of Good Posture:

- **Spinal Health:** Proper posture supports the natural curvature of the spine, reducing the risk of conditions like kyphosis or lordosis.

- **Muscle Engagement:** Maintaining good posture engages and strengthens the core, back, and shoulder muscles, contributing to overall stability.

- **Enhanced Breathing:** Correct posture allows for optimal lung capacity, improving respiratory function and oxygen intake.

- **Joint Alignment:** Proper posture ensures proper alignment of joints, reducing the risk of wear and tear on the musculoskeletal system.

- **Confidence and Self-Esteem:** Good posture not only benefits physical health but also contributes to a confident and positive self-image.

Chair Yoga Poses for Improved Posture:

1. **Mountain Pose (Tadasana Variation):**

- Sit tall in the chair with feet flat on the ground.

- Extend arms overhead, palms facing each other.

- Engage the core and lift through the spine, mimicking the standing Mountain Pose.

2. **Seated Cat-Cow Stretch:**

- Sit at the edge of the chair with hands on knees.

- Inhale, arching the back (Cow), and exhale, rounding the spine (Cat).

- Repeat to promote flexibility and alignment in the spine.

3. **Seated Twist:**

- Sit with feet flat on the ground.

- Twist the torso to one side, holding onto the back of the chair.

- Repeat on the other side, promoting spinal mobility and flexibility.

4. **Seated Forward Bend:**

- Sit at the edge of the chair with feet flat.

- Hinge at the hips and reach towards the toes, elongating the spine.

- Hold to stretch the hamstrings and promote a straight back.

5. **Chair Dandasana (Staff Pose):**

- Sit with legs extended and feet flexed.

- Place hands on the sides of the chair, lift through the spine, engaging the core.

- This pose promotes a straight and elongated posture.

6. **Seated Side Stretch:**

- Sit tall and reach one arm overhead, bending to the side.

- Feel the stretch along the side body and repeat on the

other side.

7. **Seated Warrior (Virabhadrasana Variation):**
   - Sit at the edge of the chair, extend one leg back, and bend the other knee.
   - Reach arms overhead, engaging the core and lengthening the spine.
   - Switch legs to work both sides evenly.

8. **Chair Tadasana (Chair Mountain Pose):**
   - Sit tall with feet hip-width apart.
   - Press feet into the ground, engaging leg muscles.
   - Reach arms overhead, palms facing each other.

9. **Eagle Arms (Garudasana Arms):**
   - Sit tall, cross one arm over the other, and bring palms together.
   - Lift elbows, feeling a stretch between the shoulder blades.

10. **Seated Warrior II:**
    - Sit at the edge of the chair, extend one leg back, and bend the other knee.
    - Open arms to the sides, gazing over the front hand.

Variations and Adaptations:
   - **Use of Props:** Incorporate props like blocks or cushions to support the body and facilitate proper alignment.
   - **Gentle Modifications:** Seniors with specific health concerns or limitations can make gentle modifications to poses, ensuring comfort and safety.
   - **Chair Support:** Hold onto the back or sides of the chair for added support during standing or balancing poses.

Incorporating into a Routine:

- **Consistent Practice:** Perform these chair yoga poses regularly, aiming for at least 10-15 minutes daily.

- **Mindful Awareness:** Focus on body awareness during each pose, paying attention to spinal alignment and muscle engagement.

- **Breath Coordination:** Coordinate breath with movement, inhaling to lengthen the spine and exhaling to deepen into the stretch.

Conclusion:

In conclusion, chair yoga poses for improved posture offer a tailored approach for seniors above 60 to enhance spinal alignment, flexibility, and overall body awareness. By incorporating these poses into a daily routine, individuals can reap the benefits of better posture, fostering physical well-being, and cultivating a positive self-image. This comprehensive guide serves as a roadmap for seniors looking to embark on a journey towards improved posture through the gentle and accessible practice of chair yoga.

CHAPTER 6: BUILDING STRENGTH AND STABILITY THROUGH SEATED ASANAS

Chair yoga, with its gentle yet effective approach, stands as an excellent avenue for individuals above 60 to build strength and stability. This detailed exploration delves into the significance of strength and stability, the benefits of seated asanas, and a comprehensive guide to specific poses that target these key elements. By focusing on the integration of seated asanas into a chair yoga practice, seniors can experience enhanced physical resilience, improved muscle tone, and a heightened sense of balance.

Importance of Strength and Stability:

- **Functional Independence:** Strength and stability are foundational for maintaining everyday activities, promoting independence in daily life.

- **Fall Prevention:** Building strength in the lower body and core, combined with improved stability, plays a crucial role in preventing falls, a significant concern for seniors.

- **Enhanced Joint Support:** Strong muscles provide better support to joints, reducing the risk of discomfort and potential injuries associated with weakened muscles.

- **Improved Posture:** A strong core contributes to better posture, alleviating strain on the spine and promoting overall musculoskeletal health.

- **Mental Well-being:** Physical strength and stability contribute to increased confidence and a positive self-image, influencing mental well-being.

Seated Asanas for Building Strength and Stability:

1. **Seated Leg Lifts:**
   - Sit at the edge of the chair with feet flat on the ground.
   - Lift one leg at a time, engaging the quadriceps and core muscles.
   - Gradually increase the height of the leg lifts as strength improves.

2. **Chair Squats:**
   - Stand in front of the chair with feet hip-width apart.
   - Lower into a seated position, as if sitting back into the chair, and then stand back up.
   - Repeat to strengthen the quadriceps, hamstrings, and glutes.

3. **Seated Knee Extensions:**
   - Sit tall with knees bent at a 90-degree angle.
   - Extend one leg at a time, engaging the thigh muscles.
   - Hold briefly and lower the leg, alternating sides.

4. **Seated Marching:**
   - Sit tall and lift one knee at a time in a marching motion.
   - Engage the core and maintain an upright posture.

5. **Chair Warrior I:**
   - Sit at the edge of the chair, extend one leg back, and bend the other knee.
   - Raise arms overhead, engaging the core and leg muscles.
   - Switch sides to work both legs evenly.

6. **Seated Side Leg Lifts:**
   - Sit at the edge of the chair with one leg extended to the side.

- Lift the extended leg, engaging the outer hip muscles.
- Lower and repeat on the other side.

7. **Chair Plank:**
   - Sit at the edge of the chair and place hands on the seat, fingers pointing forward.
   - Walk feet back until the body forms a straight line.
   - Hold for a few seconds, engaging the core and arm muscles.

8. **Seated Boat Pose:**
   - Sit at the edge of the chair, lean back slightly, and lift the legs, forming a V shape.
   - Engage the core and balance on the sitting bones.

9. **Seated Twist with Resistance:**
   - Hold a resistance band with both hands.
   - Sit tall and twist the torso to one side while resisting with the band.
   - Repeat on the other side to strengthen the obliques.

10. **Seated Bicep Curls:**
    - Hold light weights or water bottles in each hand.
    - Sit tall and perform bicep curls, engaging the arm muscles.

Guidelines for Building Strength and Stability:

- **Gradual Progression:** Start with a manageable number of repetitions and gradually increase as strength improves.
- **Consistency:** Perform these seated asanas regularly, aiming for at least three sessions per week.
- **Focus on Form:** Emphasize proper form and alignment to maximize the effectiveness of each exercise and

minimize the risk of injury.

- **Listen to the Body:** Pay attention to any discomfort or strain and modify exercises accordingly. Always consult a healthcare professional before beginning a new exercise routine.

Incorporating into a Routine:

- **Warm-up:** Begin with a gentle warm-up, such as neck stretches and seated cat-cow, to prepare the body for strength-building poses.

- **Structured Sequence:** Create a structured sequence that targets different muscle groups, ensuring a balanced approach to strength and stability.

- **Cool Down:** Conclude the session with a cool-down, incorporating stretches to relax and lengthen the muscles.

Conclusion:

In conclusion, building strength and stability through seated asanas in chair yoga is a powerful strategy for seniors above 60 to enhance physical resilience and overall well-being. By incorporating these specific poses into a chair yoga routine, individuals can experience the transformative benefits of increased muscle tone, improved balance, and a heightened sense of strength that positively impacts both body and mind. This comprehensive guide serves as a roadmap for seniors seeking to embark on a journey toward greater strength and stability through the accessible and beneficial practice of chair yoga.

CHAPTER 7: GENTLE CHAIR TWISTS FOR SPINAL HEALTH

Spinal health is paramount for overall well-being, especially for individuals above 60 who may face the challenges of age-related stiffness or discomfort. Gentle chair twists in the realm of chair yoga emerge as a therapeutic and accessible solution to nurture spinal flexibility, improve circulation, and alleviate tension. This detailed exploration dives into the significance of spinal health, the benefits of gentle chair twists, and provides an extensive guide to specific twists that cater to the unique needs of seniors.

Importance of Spinal Health:

- **Flexibility and Mobility:** A supple spine supports fluid movement, enhances flexibility, and contributes to overall mobility.

- **Pain Prevention:** Maintaining spinal health helps prevent discomfort and pain associated with conditions such as stiffness, arthritis, or herniated discs.

- **Improved Posture:** A healthy spine plays a pivotal role in supporting good posture, reducing strain on the back, neck, and shoulders.

- **Circulation Enhancement:** Twisting poses stimulate blood flow to the spine, nourishing the discs and supporting optimal spinal function.

- **Stress Reduction:** Gentle twists can have a calming effect on the nervous system, promoting relaxation and stress reduction.

Benefits of Gentle Chair Twists:

1. **Enhanced Spinal Flexibility:**

- Gentle chair twists target the thoracic and lumbar spine, promoting increased flexibility and range of motion.

2. **Improved Digestion:**

- Twisting poses can massage the abdominal organs, aiding digestion and promoting a healthy gut.

3. **Release of Tension:**

- Chair twists help release tension in the muscles surrounding the spine, providing relief from stiffness and discomfort.

4. **Stimulation of Internal Organs:**

- Twists stimulate internal organs, promoting better organ function and overall well-being.

5. **Encouragement of Detoxification:**

- The twisting action may aid in the detoxification process by stimulating the lymphatic system.

6. **Balancing the Nervous System:**

- Gentle twists help balance the sympathetic and parasympathetic nervous systems, fostering a sense of equilibrium.

Gentle Chair Twists Guide:

1. **Seated Spinal Twist:**

- Sit tall in the chair with feet flat on the ground.
- Inhale to lengthen the spine, and exhale to twist gently to one side.
- Hold for 15-30 seconds, breathing deeply.
- Repeat on the other side.

2. **Chair Half Twist:**

- Sit at the edge of the chair with feet flat.
- Place one hand on the opposite knee and twist gently.

- Hold for 15-20 seconds, then switch sides.

3. **Seated Eagle Twist:**
    - Cross one leg over the other at the knee.
    - Bring the opposite elbow to the outside of the crossed knee, twisting the torso.
    - Hold for 20 seconds, then switch sides.

4. **Chair Revolved Head-to-Knee Pose:**
    - Sit with legs extended and feet flexed.
    - Inhale to lengthen the spine, then exhale to twist toward one leg, bringing the opposite elbow to the outside of the knee.
    - Hold for 20 seconds and switch sides.

5. **Seated Twist with Arm Reach:**
    - Sit tall and twist the torso to one side.
    - Reach the opposite arm across the body, engaging the stretch.
    - Hold for 15-30 seconds and repeat on the other side.

6. **Chair Pigeon Twist:**
    - Sit with one ankle crossed over the opposite knee.
    - Twist the torso toward the crossed knee, feeling the stretch in the hip and lower back.
    - Hold for 20 seconds and switch sides.

7. **Supported Twist with Chair Back:**
    - Sit sideways on the chair with one hip against the backrest.
    - Hold onto the backrest and twist gently to one side.
    - Hold for 15-30 seconds, then switch sides.

8. **Seated Crescent Moon Twist:**

- Sit tall with legs extended.
- Inhale and lift arms overhead, then exhale and twist to one side, reaching one hand to the floor.
- Hold for 15-20 seconds and repeat on the other side.

Tips for Practicing Gentle Chair Twists:

- **Smooth Transitions:** Move into and out of twists slowly and with control to avoid strain.
- **Breath Awareness:** Coordinate breath with movement, inhaling to lengthen the spine and exhaling to deepen into the twist.
- **Comfortable Alignment:** Ensure that the chair provides a comfortable and stable base for the twists, adjusting as needed.
- **Listen to the Body:** Pay attention to any discomfort or strain, and modify or skip poses accordingly.

Incorporating into a Routine:

- **Warm-up:** Begin with a gentle warm-up, incorporating neck stretches, seated cat-cow, and shoulder rolls to prepare the body for twists.
- **Structured Sequence:** Design a structured sequence that includes a variety of twists to target different areas of the spine.
- **Cool Down:** Conclude the session with a cool-down, focusing on gentle stretches and relaxation.

Conclusion:

In conclusion, integrating gentle chair twists into a chair yoga practice offers a therapeutic and accessible approach to nurturing spinal health for individuals above 60. By incorporating these specific twists into a regular routine, seniors can experience the transformative benefits of improved flexibility, reduced tension, and enhanced overall well-being. This comprehensive guide serves as a valuable resource for those seeking to embark on a journey toward better spinal health through the gentle and beneficial practice of chair yoga twists.

CHAPTER 8: OPENING UP YOUR HIPS WITH SEATED STRETCHES

Hips, being a complex and vital joint, play a crucial role in the overall well-being of individuals, particularly for those above 60. Sedentary lifestyles, aging, and other factors can contribute to tightness and discomfort in the hip region. Seated stretches in the realm of chair yoga emerge as a gentle yet effective solution to alleviate tension, improve flexibility, and promote hip health. This detailed exploration delves into the importance of hip flexibility, the benefits of seated stretches, and provides an extensive guide to specific stretches designed to open up the hips.

Importance of Hip Flexibility:

- **Enhanced Range of Motion:** Flexible hips contribute to an increased range of motion, facilitating smoother and more comfortable movements.

- **Improved Posture:** Flexible hips support proper alignment of the spine, contributing to better posture and reduced strain on the lower back.

- **Alleviation of Discomfort:** Seated stretches can help alleviate tension in the hip area, reducing discomfort associated with tight muscles and joints.

- **Balance and Stability:** Flexible hips enhance balance and stability, crucial aspects for maintaining functional independence, especially as individuals age.

- **Prevention of Injury:** Flexible hips are less prone to injuries, as the joints and surrounding muscles can adapt to various movements more effectively.

Benefits of Seated Hip Stretches:

1. **Alleviation of Lower Back Pain:**

- Seated hip stretches target the muscles surrounding the hips and lower back, providing relief from discomfort associated with lumbar issues.

2. **Improved Circulation:**

- Opening up the hips enhances blood flow to the pelvic region, promoting better circulation and nourishment to the hip joints.

3. **Stress Reduction:**

- The release of tension in the hips through seated stretches can have a calming effect on the nervous system, contributing to stress reduction.

4. **Enhanced Flexibility:**

- Consistent practice of seated hip stretches gradually improves flexibility in the hip joints and surrounding muscles.

5. **Pelvic Floor Health:**

- Seated stretches engage and strengthen the pelvic floor muscles, supporting pelvic health, particularly beneficial for women.

6. **Improved Gait and Walking Comfort:**

- Flexible hips contribute to a smoother gait and walking pattern, enhancing overall comfort during daily activities.

Seated Hip Stretches Guide:

1. **Seated Knee-to-Chest Stretch:**

- Sit tall in the chair and bring one knee toward the chest.
- Hold the knee with both hands, feeling a gentle stretch in the hip.
- Hold for 20-30 seconds and switch legs.

2. **Seated Pigeon Pose:**

- Cross one ankle over the opposite knee while sitting.
- Gently press down on the crossed knee, feeling a stretch in the outer hip.
- Hold for 20-30 seconds and switch sides.

3. **Seated Figure Four Stretch:**

- Sit tall and cross one ankle over the opposite knee, forming a figure four shape.
- Lean forward slightly, feeling a stretch in the hip.
- Hold for 20-30 seconds and switch legs.

4. **Seated Hip Opener:**

- Sit with feet flat on the ground and knees bent.
- Allow the knees to fall open to the sides, feeling a stretch in the inner thighs and hips.
- Hold for 30 seconds, gradually increasing the duration.

5. **Seated Butterfly Stretch:**

- Sit tall with the soles of the feet together, allowing the knees to fall outward.
- Hold the feet and gently press down on the knees, feeling a stretch in the hips.
- Hold for 20-30 seconds.

6. **Seated Hip Flexor Stretch:**

- Sit at the edge of the chair with one foot on the ground and the other ankle crossed over the knee.
- Lean forward slightly, feeling a stretch in the hip flexor.
- Hold for 20-30 seconds and switch legs.

7. **Seated Wide-Legged Stretch:**

- Sit with legs extended wide apart.

- Lean forward, reaching towards one foot at a time, feeling a stretch in the inner thighs and hips.
- Hold for 20-30 seconds.

8. Seated Half Moon Stretch:

- Sit tall with one leg extended straight and the other foot crossed over the extended leg.
- Reach the arm on the same side as the extended leg towards the foot, feeling a stretch along the side of the hip.
- Hold for 20-30 seconds and switch sides.

Tips for Practicing Seated Hip Stretches:

- **Mindful Breathing:** Coordinate breath with movement, inhaling deeply to prepare for the stretch and exhaling to deepen into it.
- **Gentle Progression:** Gradually ease into each stretch, avoiding sudden or forceful movements to prevent injury.
- **Comfortable Alignment:** Ensure that the chair provides a stable and comfortable base for the stretches, adjusting as needed.
- **Listen to the Body:** Pay attention to sensations in the hips, and modify or skip stretches that cause discomfort.

Incorporating into a Routine:

- **Warm-up:** Begin with a gentle warm-up, incorporating seated cat-cow stretches and hip circles to prepare the body for deeper stretches.
- **Structured Sequence:** Design a structured sequence that includes a variety of seated hip stretches to target different areas of the hips.
- **Cool Down:** Conclude the session with a cool-down, focusing on gentle stretches for the entire body and

relaxation.

Conclusion:

In conclusion, opening up your hips with seated stretches in chair yoga is a nurturing and accessible approach for individuals above 60 to enhance hip flexibility, alleviate tension, and promote overall hip health. By incorporating these specific stretches into a regular routine, seniors can experience the transformative benefits of improved range of motion, reduced discomfort, and heightened well-being. This comprehensive guide serves as a valuable resource for those seeking to embark on a journey toward better hip health through the gentle and beneficial practice of seated hip stretches.

CHAPTER 9: CHAIR YOGA FOR ENHANCED BALANCE AND COORDINATION

Maintaining balance and coordination is a critical aspect of overall well-being, especially for individuals above the age of 60. Chair yoga, with its gentle and accessible approach, emerges as an effective tool for enhancing these essential elements. This detailed exploration delves into the importance of balance and coordination, the benefits of chair yoga in this context, and provides an extensive guide to specific poses and practices designed to promote stability and coordination.

Importance of Balance and Coordination:

- **Fall Prevention:** Enhanced balance reduces the risk of falls, a significant concern for seniors, preventing potential injuries and fractures.

- **Functional Independence:** Good balance and coordination support daily activities, promoting functional independence in various aspects of life.

- **Joint Health:** Improved coordination contributes to better joint health, reducing wear and tear on the musculoskeletal system.

- **Enhanced Mobility:** A well-coordinated body moves more efficiently, contributing to improved mobility and agility.

- **Postural Stability:** Balance and coordination play a crucial role in maintaining proper posture, preventing strain on the spine and supporting overall musculoskeletal health.

Benefits of Chair Yoga for Balance and Coordination:

1. **Accessible Exercise:**
   - Chair yoga provides a safe and accessible form of exercise, making it suitable for individuals with varying levels of mobility and fitness.

2. **Gentle Strength Building:**
   - Many chair yoga poses engage muscles that support balance, gradually building strength without putting excessive strain on joints.

3. **Focus on Alignment:**
   - Chair yoga emphasizes proper alignment, helping individuals develop body awareness, a key component of balance.

4. **Mind-Body Connection:**
   - The mindful approach of chair yoga fosters a strong mind-body connection, enhancing coordination and proprioception.

5. **Improvement in Reaction Time:**
   - Practicing chair yoga can enhance reaction time, a crucial factor in preventing falls and maintaining coordination.

6. **Relaxation and Stress Reduction:**
   - The relaxation component of chair yoga contributes to stress reduction, positively influencing overall mental and physical well-being.

Chair Yoga Poses for Enhanced Balance and Coordination:

1. **Seated Mountain Pose:**
   - Sit tall with feet flat on the ground.
   - Ground through the feet, engage the core, and reach arms overhead.

- Hold for 20-30 seconds, focusing on a stable and aligned posture.

2. **Seated Tree Pose:**

  - Sit with spine tall and lift one foot, placing the sole against the inner thigh or calf of the opposite leg.
  - Bring hands to heart center and hold for 20-30 seconds.
  - Switch legs and repeat.

3. **Seated Warrior III:**

  - Sit at the edge of the chair and extend one leg straight back while reaching arms forward.
  - Engage the core for stability and hold for 20-30 seconds.
  - Switch legs and repeat.

4. **Chair Squats:**

  - Stand in front of the chair with feet hip-width apart.
  - Lower into a seated position, as if sitting back into the chair, and then stand back up.
  - Repeat to build strength and coordination.

5. **Seated Side Leg Lifts:**

  - Sit tall with one leg extended to the side.
  - Lift the extended leg, engaging the outer hip muscles.
  - Lower and repeat for both sides.

6. **Seated Twist with Arm Reach:**

  - Sit tall and twist the torso to one side.
  - Reach the opposite arm across the body, engaging the stretch.
  - Hold for 20-30 seconds and repeat on the other side.

7. **Seated Half Moon Stretch:**

  - Sit tall with one leg extended straight and the other foot crossed over the extended leg.

- Reach the arm on the same side as the extended leg towards the foot, feeling a stretch along the side of the hip.

- Hold for 20-30 seconds and switch sides.

8. **Seated Figure Eight Arm Movements:**

- Sit tall and extend arms to the sides.

- Move arms in a figure-eight pattern, coordinating movement with breath.

- This practice enhances coordination and focus.

Guidelines for Practicing Chair Yoga for Balance and Coordination:

- **Steady Breathing:** Maintain steady and controlled breathing throughout each pose, using breath to enhance focus and stability.

- **Consistent Practice:** Incorporate chair yoga for balance and coordination into a regular routine, aiming for at least 10-15 minutes daily.

- **Mindful Transitions:** Pay attention to transitions between poses, ensuring controlled movements to build awareness and coordination.

- **Use of Props:** Utilize props, such as a sturdy chair, for support and stability, gradually reducing reliance as confidence and strength increase.

Incorporating into a Routine:

- **Warm-up:** Begin with a gentle warm-up, incorporating neck stretches, shoulder rolls, and seated cat-cow stretches to prepare the body for balance-focused poses.

- **Structured Sequence:** Design a structured sequence that includes a variety of chair yoga poses for balance and coordination, progressing from simpler to more challenging poses.

- **Cool Down:** Conclude the session with a cool-down, focusing on gentle stretches and relaxation to promote a sense of calm.

Conclusion:

In conclusion, chair yoga for enhanced balance and coordination provides a gentle yet powerful approach for individuals above 60 to improve stability and overall well-being. By incorporating these specific poses and practices into a regular routine, seniors can experience the transformative benefits of increased coordination, enhanced balance, and a heightened sense of body awareness. This comprehensive guide serves as a valuable resource for those seeking to embark on a journey toward improved balance and coordination through the accessible and beneficial practice of chair yoga.

CHAPTER 10: BREATHING TECHNIQUES FOR RELAXATION AND STRESS REDUCTION

In the fast-paced world we live in, finding effective methods to manage stress and promote relaxation is crucial for maintaining overall well-being. One powerful and accessible tool that individuals of all ages can incorporate into their daily lives is the practice of intentional breathing techniques. This comprehensive exploration delves into the physiological and psychological benefits of conscious breathing, different types of breathing techniques, and practical guidance on incorporating these practices for relaxation and stress reduction.

The Science Behind Breathing and Stress:

Understanding the intricate connection between breathing and stress response is foundational to appreciating the effectiveness of breathing techniques for relaxation. The autonomic nervous system, comprised of the sympathetic and parasympathetic branches, plays a central role in regulating our body's responses to stress. The sympathetic nervous system, often referred to as the "fight or flight" response, is activated during times of stress or danger, leading to increased heart rate, shallow breathing, and heightened alertness. On the contrary, the parasympathetic nervous system, known as the "rest and digest" response, promotes relaxation, slowing the heart rate, and deepening the breath.

Benefits of Conscious Breathing:

- **Stress Reduction:** Conscious breathing activates the parasympathetic nervous system, countering the effects of stress and promoting a sense of calm.

- **Improved Mental Clarity:** Deep, intentional breaths increase oxygen flow to the brain, enhancing cognitive function and mental clarity.

- **Enhanced Emotional Regulation:** Breathing techniques can assist in managing emotions by creating a pause and promoting a more thoughtful response to challenging situations.

- **Muscle Relaxation:** Deep breathing helps release tension in the muscles, reducing physical symptoms of stress like headaches and muscle stiffness.

- **Lowered Blood Pressure:** Practicing conscious breathing has been linked to lower blood pressure, contributing to cardiovascular health.

- **Improved Sleep Quality:** Incorporating breathing exercises into a bedtime routine can help calm the mind and improve sleep quality.

Common Breathing Techniques for Relaxation:

1. Diaphragmatic Breathing (Deep Belly Breathing):

- Sit or lie down in a comfortable position.

- Place one hand on the chest and the other on the abdomen.

- Inhale deeply through the nose, allowing the abdomen to expand.

- Exhale slowly through pursed lips, feeling the abdomen fall.

- Repeat for several breath cycles.

2. 4-7-8 Breathing (Relaxing Breath):

- Inhale quietly through the nose for a count of 4.

- Hold the breath for a count of 7.

- Exhale completely through the mouth for a count of 8.

- Repeat for several cycles, gradually increasing duration.

3. **Alternate Nostril Breathing (Nadi Shodhana):**
   - Sit comfortably with a straight spine.
   - Use the right thumb to close the right nostril and inhale through the left nostril.
   - Close the left nostril with the right ring finger, release the right nostril, and exhale.
   - Inhale through the right nostril, close it, release the left nostril, and exhale.
   - Repeat for several cycles, promoting balance and relaxation.

4. **Box Breathing (Square Breathing):**
   - Inhale through the nose for a count of 4.
   - Hold the breath for a count of 4.
   - Exhale through the mouth for a count of 4.
   - Pause for a count of 4 before inhaling again.
   - Repeat for several breath cycles.

5. **Guided Imagery Breathing:**
   - Close the eyes and visualize a peaceful scene.
   - Inhale deeply, imagining the scent of the surroundings.
   - Exhale slowly, envisioning tension leaving the body.
   - Combine deep breathing with a calming mental image for relaxation.

Practical Guidance for Incorporating Breathing Techniques:

- **Consistency is Key:** Establish a regular practice by incorporating breathing exercises into daily routines. Aim for at least 5-10 minutes of focused breathing each day.
- **Mindful Awareness:** During breathing exercises,

cultivate mindful awareness by focusing on the sensation of the breath. This anchors the mind to the present moment.

- **Adapt to Your Comfort:** Choose a breathing technique that resonates with you. Experiment with different methods to find what feels most comfortable and effective.

- **Combine Breathing with Activities:** Integrate conscious breathing into daily activities, such as while commuting, working at a desk, or waiting in line. This fosters a seamless incorporation into daily life.

- **Use Visual and Auditory Aids:** Enhance the experience by incorporating soothing visuals or calming sounds. This can include nature sounds, calming music, or guided meditation apps.

- **Set Intentions:** Before beginning a breathing session, set intentions or affirmations. This creates a positive mental space and enhances the impact of the practice.

Incorporating Breathwork into a Relaxation Routine:

- **Preparation:** Find a quiet and comfortable space to sit or lie down.

- **Body Scan:** Perform a brief body scan, noticing areas of tension or discomfort.

- **Choose a Technique:** Select a breathing technique that aligns with your preferences and goals for the session.

- **Guided Session:** Use guided meditation apps or recordings for structured sessions led by experienced instructors.

- **Mindful Focus:** Direct your attention to the breath, observing its rhythm and sensations.

- **Progressive Relaxation:** Combine breathwork with progressive muscle relaxation, releasing tension from head to toe.

- **Closing Reflection:** Conclude the session with a moment of reflection, expressing gratitude or acknowledging positive aspects of your experience.

Conclusion:

In conclusion, conscious breathing techniques for relaxation and stress reduction offer a simple yet profound avenue for individuals seeking to manage the demands of modern life. By understanding the physiological mechanisms at play and exploring various breathing techniques, individuals can tailor their practices to suit their needs. Incorporating intentional breathwork into daily routines empowers individuals to cultivate a sense of calm, enhance mental clarity, and build resilience in the face of stressors. This comprehensive guide serves as a valuable resource for those embarking on a journey toward greater relaxation and well-being through the transformative power of breath.

CHAPTER 11: INCORPORATING MEDITATION INTO YOUR DAILY CHAIR YOGA ROUTINE

Meditation, a practice rooted in ancient traditions, has gained widespread recognition for its profound impact on mental, emotional, and physical well-being. When combined with chair yoga, a gentle and accessible form of exercise, meditation becomes a powerful tool for fostering holistic mind-body wellness. This detailed exploration delves into the synergistic benefits of combining meditation and chair yoga, the various meditation techniques suitable for a seated practice, and practical guidance on seamlessly integrating meditation into your daily chair yoga routine.

The Synergy of Meditation and Chair Yoga:

- **Mindful Movement:** Chair yoga involves gentle, intentional movements that encourage mindfulness. Combining meditation enhances this mindfulness, allowing for a deeper connection between body and mind.

- **Enhanced Relaxation:** Both meditation and chair yoga individually promote relaxation. When intertwined, they create a harmonious synergy, amplifying the overall sense of calm and tranquility.

- **Stress Reduction:** Meditation's ability to calm the mind complements chair yoga's stress-relieving physical movements, providing a comprehensive approach to stress reduction.

- **Improved Focus:** Meditation cultivates mental clarity and focus, which can enhance the effectiveness of chair yoga poses by fostering a deeper mind-body connection.

- **Holistic Wellness:** The combination of meditation and chair yoga supports holistic wellness by addressing both the physical and mental aspects of well-being.

Meditation Techniques for a Seated Practice:

1. **Mindfulness Meditation:**

   - Sit comfortably in a chair, focusing on the breath or a chosen point of attention.

   - Gently bring the mind back to the present moment when distractions arise.

   - Start with short sessions and gradually extend the duration.

2. **Loving-Kindness Meditation (Metta):**

   - Cultivate feelings of compassion and love towards oneself and others.

   - Repeat phrases such as "May I (or others) be happy, may I (or others) be healthy, may I (or others) be safe, may I (or others) be at ease."

3. **Body Scan Meditation:**

   - Progressively bring awareness to different parts of the body, starting from the toes and moving up to the head.

   - Notice sensations without judgment, allowing for relaxation and release of tension.

4. **Guided Visualization:**

   - Use guided imagery to create a mental picture of a peaceful and serene place.

   - Imagine details like colors, sounds, and sensations, engaging the senses for a deeper experience.

5. **Breath Awareness Meditation:**

   - Focus on the natural flow of the breath.

- Notice the inhalation and exhalation, observing the sensations in the nose, chest, or abdomen.
- Use the breath as an anchor to stay present.

6. Mantra Meditation:

- Choose a word, phrase, or sound as a mantra.
- Repeat the mantra silently or aloud, allowing it to occupy the mind and create a meditative state.

7. Counting Breath Meditation:

- Inhale and exhale naturally, counting each breath cycle.
- Start with a count of 1 and gradually increase to 10.
- If the mind wanders, return to 1 and restart the counting.

Practical Guidance for Integration:

- **Set a Consistent Schedule:** Choose a specific time each day to integrate meditation into your chair yoga routine, creating a consistent and dedicated practice.
- **Create a Comfortable Space:** Designate a quiet and comfortable space for your practice. Ensure your chair is supportive and allows for an upright yet relaxed posture.
- **Start with Short Sessions:** Begin with shorter meditation sessions, gradually increasing the duration as you become more comfortable with the practice.
- **Seamless Transitions:** Integrate meditation seamlessly into your chair yoga routine by starting with a few minutes of focused breathing before moving into yoga poses.
- **Combine Movement and Stillness:** Alternate between chair yoga poses and periods of stillness or meditation. This combination offers a dynamic yet balanced approach to mind-body wellness.
- **Use Guided Resources:** Leverage guided meditation

apps, videos, or recordings to enhance your practice. Expert-led sessions can provide structure and guidance, especially for beginners.

- **Combine Meditation Techniques**: Experiment with different meditation techniques to discover what resonates best with you. A combination of mindfulness, loving-kindness, and visualization can add variety to your routine.

Sequencing Your Daily Chair Yoga Routine with Meditation:

- **Begin with Centering Breaths:**
    - Sit comfortably and focus on a few rounds of diaphragmatic breathing to center the mind and body.

- **Mindful Movement with Chair Yoga Poses:**
    - Flow into your chair yoga routine, moving through gentle poses with awareness and intentional breathing.

- **Transitional Breathwork:**
    - Pause between poses for a few moments of intentional breathwork, promoting a seamless transition from movement to stillness.

- **Meditative Seated Posture:**
    - Find a comfortable seated position in the chair, ensuring an upright spine.
    - Choose a meditation technique (e.g., mindfulness or loving-kindness) and practice for 5-10 minutes.

- **Transition to Guided Visualization:**
    - Incorporate a guided visualization meditation, immersing yourself in a serene mental landscape.

- **Closing Reflection:**
    - Conclude the session with a few moments

of gratitude or reflection, acknowledging the benefits of your combined chair yoga and meditation practice.

Conclusion:

In conclusion, incorporating meditation into your daily chair yoga routine offers a holistic and transformative approach to mind-body wellness. The synergy of mindful movement and intentional stillness creates a powerful combination that nurtures physical health, mental clarity, and emotional well-being. By exploring different meditation techniques, establishing a consistent practice, and seamlessly integrating meditation into your chair yoga routine, you embark on a journey toward a more balanced and harmonious life. This comprehensive guide serves as a valuable resource for those seeking to enrich their chair yoga practice with the profound benefits of meditation.

CHAPTER 12: EXPLORING MINDFULNESS THROUGH SEATED POSES

Mindfulness, rooted in ancient contemplative traditions, has become a widely recognized and embraced practice for cultivating a heightened state of awareness and presence. When infused into seated yoga poses, this practice takes on a transformative quality, inviting individuals to explore the richness of the present moment while promoting physical, mental, and emotional well-being. This detailed exploration delves into the essence of mindfulness, the benefits of integrating it into seated yoga poses, and a comprehensive guide to practicing mindfulness in a seated posture for a holistic approach to self-discovery.

Understanding Mindfulness:

Mindfulness, at its core, involves intentionally paying attention to the present moment without judgment. It is a state of heightened awareness that encompasses observing thoughts, feelings, bodily sensations, and the surrounding environment. Cultivating mindfulness involves bringing one's full attention to the current experience, allowing for a deepening connection with the unfolding reality. By being fully present, individuals can navigate the complexities of life with clarity, equanimity, and a sense of purpose.

Benefits of Mindfulness in Seated Poses:

- **Stress Reduction:** Mindfulness promotes a relaxation response, reducing stress hormones and fostering a sense of calm in seated poses.

- **Enhanced Body Awareness:** Seated poses offer an opportunity to tune into the body's sensations, promoting a deeper understanding of physical well-being.

- **Improved Posture:** Mindfulness encourages awareness of body alignment, supporting the maintenance of an upright and comfortable seated posture.

- **Emotional Regulation:** Through seated mindfulness, individuals can observe and regulate emotions, fostering emotional intelligence and resilience.

- **Increased Concentration:** The practice of mindfulness sharpens attention and concentration, which can be beneficial for both the seated pose and daily life.

- **Cultivation of Inner Peace:** Mindfulness in seated poses allows for the cultivation of inner peace, creating a refuge within oneself.

Guide to Exploring Mindfulness in Seated Poses:

1. Mindful Breathing in Seated Meditation:

- Find a comfortable seated position with an upright spine.

- Direct attention to the breath, noticing the inhalation and exhalation.

- Allow the breath to be a focal point, gently guiding the mind back when distractions arise.

2. Body Scan Meditation in Seated Pose:

- Start from the toes and gradually shift attention through each part of the body.

- Observe sensations without judgment, fostering a connection with the body.

3. Mindful Observation in Seated Stillness:

- Choose a point of focus, such as a candle flame or an object.

- Observe the chosen point mindfully, noticing details,

colors, and shapes.

4. **Mindful Eating in a Seated Pose:**

- Incorporate mindfulness into seated meals, paying full attention to the sensory experience of eating.
- Notice flavors, textures, and the act of chewing with intention.

5. **Loving-Kindness Meditation in Seated Posture:**

- Begin with focusing on sending loving-kindness to oneself.
- Extend these wishes to others, gradually expanding the circle of compassion.

6. **Seated Yoga Poses with Mindful Awareness:**

- Engage in seated yoga poses mindfully, observing the body's sensations and any areas of tension.
- Bring attention to the breath while moving through seated poses.

7. **Mindful Journaling in a Seated Position:**

- Sit comfortably with a journal, allowing thoughts and feelings to flow onto the pages.
- Reflect mindfully on experiences, observations, or gratitude.

8. **Guided Visualization in Seated Meditation:**

- Close the eyes and follow a guided visualization, immersing oneself in a peaceful and serene mental landscape.

Mindful Practices for Different Seated Poses:

1. **Seated Cross-Legged Pose (Sukhasana):**

- Ground through the sit bones, feeling the connection with the earth.
- Engage in mindful breathing, bringing attention to the

rise and fall of the chest or the sensation of air passing through the nostrils.

2. **Seated Hero Pose (Virasana):**

- Kneel with the sit bones resting on the floor or a cushion.
- Focus on the alignment of the spine and the sensation of stretch in the thighs.
- Observe the breath as you maintain the pose.

3. **Seated Wide-Legged Forward Fold (Upavistha Konasana):**

- Sit with legs extended wide apart.
- Hinge forward from the hips, maintaining a straight spine.
- Mindfully explore the stretch along the inner thighs and spine.

4. **Seated Spinal Twist (Ardha Matsyendrasana):**

- Sit tall and twist gently, bringing the opposite hand to the outer knee.
- Observe the twist in the spine and the breath.
- Repeat on the other side.

Tips for Enhancing Mindfulness in Seated Poses:

- **Gentle Awareness:** Approach mindfulness with gentleness and curiosity, allowing experiences to unfold without judgment.
- **Regular Practice:** Cultivate mindfulness through regular practice, gradually extending the duration as the practice deepens.
- **Create a Sacred Space:** Designate a space for seated mindfulness, free from distractions, to enhance the sense of sacredness in the practice.
- **Body-Scan Check-Ins:** Periodically check in with different parts of the body during seated poses, noting

sensations and adjusting posture mindfully.

- **Mindful Transitions:** Bring mindfulness into transitions between seated poses, maintaining awareness even in movement.

- **Utilize Guided Resources:** Explore guided meditations or mindfulness apps to provide structure and support during seated mindfulness practice.

Incorporating Mindfulness into a Daily Seated Yoga Routine:

- **Preparation:** Begin by finding a comfortable seated position, ensuring a stable and aligned posture.

- **Centering Breath:** Initiate the practice with a few rounds of centering breaths, anchoring attention to the present moment.

- **Mindful Seated Poses:** Engage in seated yoga poses with a focus on mindful awareness, incorporating breath and intentional movement.

- **Mindfulness Meditation:** Transition into seated mindfulness meditation, choosing a technique that aligns with your intention for the session.

- **Mindful Eating or Journaling:** Extend mindfulness beyond the practice by incorporating it into other daily activities, such as eating or journaling.

- **Closing Reflection:** Conclude the session with a moment of gratitude or reflection, acknowledging the benefits of exploring mindfulness through seated poses.

Conclusion:

In conclusion, exploring mindfulness through seated poses offers a transformative journey into presence, self-discovery, and holistic well-being. By infusing mindfulness into seated yoga, individuals can cultivate a heightened awareness that extends into all aspects of life. This comprehensive guide serves as a valuable resource for those seeking to embark on a journey toward mindfulness, fostering a deep connection with the present moment and unlocking the transformative potential of seated poses in yoga.

CHAPTER 13: CHAIR YOGA FOR JOINT HEALTH AND FLEXIBILITY

Chair yoga, a gentle and accessible form of yoga, serves as a remarkable tool for promoting joint health and flexibility, particularly for individuals who may face physical limitations or challenges. This comprehensive exploration delves into the significance of joint health and flexibility, the unique benefits of chair yoga in this context, and a detailed guide on specific chair yoga poses designed to enhance joint mobility and flexibility.

Understanding Joint Health and Flexibility:

1. Joint Health:

- Joints are pivotal in facilitating movement and supporting the musculoskeletal system.

- Optimal joint health is characterized by the smooth functioning of joints, minimal discomfort, and the absence of stiffness or restricted movement.

2. Flexibility:

- Flexibility refers to the ability of muscles and joints to move through their full range of motion.

- Maintaining flexibility is crucial for preventing injuries, enhancing mobility, and supporting overall physical well-being.

The Benefits of Chair Yoga for Joint Health and Flexibility:

- **Accessible Movement:** Chair yoga provides a safe and accessible way for individuals with limited mobility or physical challenges to engage in therapeutic movement.

- **Reduced Impact:** The seated nature of chair yoga minimizes impact on joints, making it suitable for those with joint concerns or conditions like arthritis.

- **Gentle Stretching:** Chair yoga incorporates gentle stretching, promoting flexibility without putting excessive strain on joints.

- **Increased Circulation:** The movements in chair yoga enhance blood circulation, supporting joint health by delivering nutrients and oxygen to the surrounding tissues.

- **Enhanced Synovial Fluid Production:** Synovial fluid lubricates joints, reducing friction and promoting smooth movement. Chair yoga stimulates the production of this vital fluid.

- **Improved Range of Motion:** Consistent practice of chair yoga poses gradually improves joint range of motion, enhancing flexibility and reducing stiffness.

- **Muscle Strengthening:** While emphasizing joint health, chair yoga also engages muscles, providing stability and support to the joints.

Chair Yoga Poses for Joint Health and Flexibility:

1. Seated Neck Stretches:

- Sit tall in the chair and gently tilt the head to one side, feeling a stretch along the neck.

- Hold for a few breaths, then repeat on the other side.

- Incorporate gentle neck circles for added mobility.

2. Seated Shoulder Rolls:

- Lift the shoulders up towards the ears, roll them back, and then down.

- Repeat this circular motion, promoting flexibility and relieving tension in the shoulders.

3. Seated Cat-Cow Stretch:

- Sit at the edge of the chair with hands on knees.

- Inhale, arch the back, and lift the chest (Cow).
- Exhale, round the spine, and tuck the chin to the chest (Cat).
- Repeat for a gentle spinal stretch.

4. Seated Side Bends:

- Inhale, lift one arm overhead, and gently bend to the side.
- Feel the stretch along the side of the body.
- Hold, then return to the center and repeat on the other side.

5. Seated Forward Fold:

- Sit tall with feet hip-width apart.
- Hinge at the hips, bringing the chest forward and reaching towards the toes.
- Hold for a few breaths, feeling the stretch in the hamstrings and lower back.

6. Ankle Circles:

- Extend one leg and rotate the ankle clockwise and then counterclockwise.
- Switch legs and repeat.
- This helps improve ankle mobility.

7. Seated Hip Opener:

- Cross one ankle over the opposite knee.
- Gently press down on the crossed knee, feeling a stretch in the hip.
- Hold, then switch to the other side.

8. Seated Knee Hug:

- Lift one knee towards the chest, hugging it with both hands.

- Hold for a moment, feeling the stretch in the hip and lower back.

- Repeat on the other side.

Guidelines for Practicing Chair Yoga for Joint Health:

- **Mindful Breathing:** Coordinate movements with breath, fostering a mindful and intentional practice.

- **Comfortable Seated Position:** Ensure a comfortable and stable seated position, using props like cushions or blankets for added support.

- **Listen to Your Body:** Pay attention to sensations and avoid pushing into discomfort. Modify poses as needed.

- **Gradual Progression:** Start with simpler poses and gradually progress to more challenging ones as joint flexibility improves.

- **Consistency is Key:** Regular practice is essential for experiencing the cumulative benefits of chair yoga for joint health.

Incorporating into a Routine:

- **Warm-up:** Begin with gentle warm-up exercises, such as neck stretches and shoulder rolls, to prepare the body for the practice.

- **Structured Sequence:** Design a structured sequence that targets different joints, ensuring a comprehensive approach to joint health.

- **Cool Down:** Conclude the session with a cool-down, incorporating relaxation poses to release any tension built up during the practice.

Conclusion:

In conclusion, chair yoga for joint health and flexibility offers a gentle yet effective approach for individuals seeking to improve mobility and reduce stiffness. By incorporating specific poses into a regular routine, individuals can experience the therapeutic benefits of enhanced joint health and flexibility. This comprehensive guide serves as a valuable resource for those embarking on a journey toward improved joint function and overall well-being through the accessible and beneficial practice of chair yoga.

CHAPTER 14: TIPS FOR ADAPTING POSES TO INDIVIDUAL ABILITIES

Yoga, with its diverse array of poses and practices, is a transformative discipline that offers numerous benefits for physical, mental, and emotional well-being. One of the key principles of yoga is adaptability, making it accessible to individuals of varying abilities, ages, and fitness levels. This comprehensive guide explores the importance of adapting yoga poses to individual abilities, the principles behind effective modifications, and practical tips for creating an inclusive and personalized yoga practice.

Understanding the Need for Adaptation:

- **Diversity of Practitioners:**
    - Yoga is practiced by individuals with diverse backgrounds, body types, and physical conditions.
    - Adapting poses ensures that yoga remains inclusive, making it accessible to everyone, regardless of age, fitness level, or physical limitations.

- **Injury Prevention and Recovery:**
    - Adapting poses is crucial for preventing injuries and supporting individuals in their recovery from injuries or chronic conditions.
    - Modifications allow practitioners to engage in yoga safely and gradually build strength and flexibility.

- **Personalization for Progress:**

- Personalizing poses based on individual abilities facilitates progress and growth.
- Modifications empower practitioners to tailor their practice to align with their unique needs and goals.

Principles of Effective Pose Adaptation:

- **Awareness of Body Limitations:**
    - Practitioners and instructors should be mindful of individual body limitations, injuries, or health conditions.
    - Personalized adaptations take into account the unique requirements and challenges each individual may face.

- **Focus on Alignment and Safety:**
    - Adaptations should prioritize proper alignment to ensure the safety of the practitioner.
    - Emphasize stability and avoid pushing the body into positions that may cause strain or discomfort.

- **Use of Props:**
    - Props, such as blocks, straps, blankets, and chairs, are valuable tools for adapting poses.
    - Props provide support, stability, and assistance, helping practitioners experience the benefits of poses more comfortably.

- **Mindful Breath and Intention:**
    - Encourage practitioners to focus on their breath and set mindful intentions during adapted poses.
    - The breath becomes a guiding force, fostering a connection between the body and mind.

- **Gradual Progression:**

- Adaptations often involve gradually progressing into a pose, allowing the body to acclimate and build strength over time.
- Encourage practitioners to be patient and embrace a gradual approach.

Tips for Adapting Specific Yoga Poses:

1. Adapting Downward-Facing Dog (Adho Mukha Svanasana):

- Use a chair or wall for support, allowing practitioners to maintain alignment while reducing weight on the wrists.
- Keep the knees slightly bent if there are concerns with flexibility or discomfort.

2. Modifying Warrior Poses (Virabhadrasana I, II, III):

- Shorten the stance for a more stable base, reducing strain on the hips and knees.
- Use a chair or wall for balance and support in Warrior III.

3. Chair Yoga Modifications:

- Chair yoga is inherently adaptive, making it suitable for individuals with limited mobility or those who prefer a seated practice.
- Incorporate seated twists, stretches, and gentle movements with the support of a chair.

4. Supported Backbends:

- Use props like bolsters or blankets to support the spine in backbends, ensuring comfort and safety.
- Gradually increase the height of the prop as flexibility improves.

5. Gentle Seated Forward Folds:

- Allow practitioners to bend the knees during seated forward folds to ease tension on the hamstrings.

- Use props to support the hands or forearms on the ground if reaching the floor is challenging.

6. Adapting Tree Pose (Vrikshasana):

- Modify by placing the foot on the inner calf or ankle instead of the thigh.

- Utilize a wall or chair for balance support.

Practical Tips for Instructors:

- **Individual Assessments:**
    - Conduct individual assessments to understand practitioners' abilities, limitations, and any specific concerns they may have.
    - Provide modifications based on this assessment to ensure a personalized practice.

- **Clear Communication:**
    - Clearly communicate pose modifications and alternatives during classes.
    - Encourage practitioners to communicate their comfort levels and ask questions.

- **Accessible Language:**
    - Use accessible language and cues that guide practitioners to make necessary adjustments.
    - Demonstrate adaptations and encourage participants to explore variations that suit their bodies.

- **Encourage Self-Exploration:**
    - Foster a sense of self-exploration and self-awareness.
    - Encourage practitioners to listen to their bodies and choose variations that feel right for them.

- **Regular Check-Ins:**
    - Conduct regular check-ins with practitioners,

especially those with specific health concerns or injuries.

- Stay informed about any changes in their physical conditions that may necessitate adjustments.

Creating an Inclusive Yoga Environment:

- **Open Communication:**
    - Create an open and non-judgmental space where practitioners feel comfortable communicating their needs.
    - Establish trust by actively listening and responding to individual concerns.

- **Diversity of Offerings:**
    - Offer a diverse range of classes, including chair yoga, restorative yoga, and gentle yoga, to cater to different abilities and preferences.

- **Educational Workshops:**
    - Conduct workshops on adapting poses, providing practitioners with the knowledge and tools to personalize their practice.

- **Community Support:**
    - Foster a sense of community support, where practitioners encourage and inspire each other in their unique yoga journeys.

- **Inclusive Language and Imagery:**
    - Use inclusive language and imagery in marketing materials, class descriptions, and verbal cues to welcome practitioners of all abilities.

Conclusion:

In conclusion, adapting yoga poses to individual abilities is a fundamental aspect of fostering inclusivity and ensuring that the transformative benefits of yoga are accessible to everyone. This comprehensive guide serves as a valuable resource for practitioners and instructors alike, offering insights into the principles of effective adaptation, practical tips for modifying specific poses, and strategies for creating an inclusive yoga environment. By embracing adaptability and personalization, yoga becomes a truly transformative practice that honors the uniqueness of each individual's journey toward holistic well-being.

CHAPTER 15: PROGRESSING YOUR PRACTICE: INTERMEDIATE CHAIR YOGA POSES

Chair yoga, known for its accessibility and gentle nature, is an ideal practice for individuals of all ages and abilities. As practitioners advance in their chair yoga journey, the exploration of intermediate poses becomes an exciting avenue for enhancing strength, flexibility, and the mind-body connection. This comprehensive guide delves into the significance of progressing your chair yoga practice, the benefits of intermediate poses, and a detailed exploration of specific postures designed to elevate your yoga experience.

Significance of Progressing in Chair Yoga:

- **Holistic Advancement:**
    - Progressing in chair yoga signifies a holistic approach to well-being, encompassing physical strength, flexibility, and mental resilience.
    - Advancement in practice reflects a deeper connection with the body, breath, and the transformative aspects of yoga.

- **Expanded Mind-Body Awareness:**
    - As practitioners progress, there is a heightened awareness of the mind-body connection.
    - Intermediate poses offer opportunities for greater concentration, mindfulness, and a profound understanding of the body's capabilities.

- **Continued Physical Benefits:**
  - Advancing to intermediate chair yoga poses provides ongoing physical benefits, including increased strength, improved joint mobility, and enhanced flexibility.
  - The practice evolves to address more intricate aspects of physical well-being.
- **Challenges and Growth:**
  - Intermediate poses introduce challenges that stimulate growth and self-discovery.
  - Overcoming challenges fosters a sense of accomplishment and encourages practitioners to explore the edges of their comfort zones.

Benefits of Intermediate Chair Yoga Poses:

- **Muscle Engagement and Strengthening:**
  - Intermediate poses involve more muscle engagement, promoting strength and toning.
  - Targeted muscle activation contributes to improved stability and overall physical resilience.
- **Enhanced Flexibility and Range of Motion:**
  - Intermediate chair yoga poses gently push the boundaries of flexibility, encouraging a broader range of motion.
  - Gradual exploration of deeper stretches contributes to increased flexibility.
- **Balancing Challenges:**
  - Many intermediate poses focus on balance, requiring practitioners to refine their stability and concentration.
  - Balancing challenges contribute to improved proprioception and coordination.

- **Deepening Mindfulness:**
  - The complexity of intermediate poses necessitates a heightened state of mindfulness.
  - Practitioners develop a deeper presence, cultivating a meditative quality in their practice.
- **Continued Joint Health:**
  - Intermediate poses continue to support joint health by encouraging movement in various directions.
  - Joint mobility is sustained, contributing to overall joint well-being.

Exploration of Intermediate Chair Yoga Poses:

1. Warrior Chair Pose:

- Sit tall in the chair, extend one leg forward, and the other leg back.
- Raise the arms overhead, palms facing each other.
- Engage the core and hold the pose, switching sides after a few breaths.
- Benefits: Strengthens the legs, improves balance, and engages the core.

2. Seated Twist with Leg Extension:

- Sit with legs extended.
- Bend one knee and cross it over the opposite leg.
- Place the opposite elbow on the outside of the bent knee and twist.
- Benefits: Enhances spinal mobility, stretches the hips, and engages the core.

3. Eagle Arms in Chair Pose:

- Sit tall, extend the arms forward, and cross one arm over

the other, wrapping them around each other.

- Lift the elbows and drop the shoulders, holding the pose.
- Benefits: Opens the shoulders, improves upper body strength, and cultivates focus.

4. **Seated Pigeon Pose:**

- Sit on the edge of the chair, cross one ankle over the opposite knee.
- Gently lean forward, keeping the back straight.
- Benefits: Stretches the hips and glutes, improves flexibility in the lower back.

5. **Chair Plank Pose:**

- Sit on the edge of the chair, place hands on the seat, and walk the feet back.
- Create a straight line from head to heels, engaging the core.
- Benefits: Strengthens the arms, shoulders, and core, improves overall body awareness.

6. **Seated Boat Pose:**

- Sit with knees bent, feet flat on the floor.
- Lean back slightly, lift the feet off the ground, and extend the legs.
- Hold the pose, engaging the core.
- Benefits: Strengthens the core, hip flexors, and promotes balance.

7. **Chair Camel Pose:**

- Sit on the chair with hands on the lower back.
- Arch the spine backward, lifting the chest and opening the heart.
- Benefits: Stretches the front body, improves spine

flexibility, and opens the chest.

8. **Seated Extended Triangle Pose:**

- Sit with legs extended wide.

- Reach one hand towards the opposite foot, keeping the spine long.

- Benefits: Stretches the sides of the body, promotes spinal flexibility.

Tips for Progressing Safely:

- **Mindful Progression:**
    - Progress at a pace that feels comfortable and safe.
    - Listen to your body, and do not push into discomfort or strain.

- **Consistent Practice:**
    - Regular, consistent practice is key to progressing in chair yoga.
    - Establishing a routine enhances muscle memory and facilitates gradual improvement.

- **Use of Props:**
    - Props such as blocks, straps, or cushions can provide additional support during intermediate poses.
    - Props assist in maintaining proper alignment and preventing strain.

- **Seek Guidance:**
    - Consider seeking guidance from a certified chair yoga instructor or physical therapist.
    - Professional guidance ensures that you are progressing appropriately and safely.

- **Warm-Up and Cool Down:**
    - Always incorporate a thorough warm-up before

attempting intermediate poses.

- ◦ Include a cool-down to release any tension built up during the practice.

Incorporating Intermediate Poses into Your Routine:

- **Start with a Warm-Up:**
  - ◦ Begin your chair yoga practice with gentle warm-up exercises to prepare the body for more challenging poses.

- **Structured Sequence:**
  - ◦ Design a structured sequence that gradually introduces intermediate poses.
  - ◦ Progress from simpler poses to more complex ones, allowing the body to adapt.

- **Balanced Practice:**
  - ◦ Ensure a balance between strength-building poses, flexibility-enhancing stretches, and relaxation.
  - ◦ A well-rounded practice addresses multiple aspects of physical and mental well-being.

- **Mindful Breathing:**
  - ◦ Incorporate mindful breathing throughout your practice to enhance focus and connection with each pose.

- **Cool Down and Relaxation:**
  - ◦ Conclude your session with a cool-down, incorporating poses that promote relaxation and release any residual tension.

Conclusion:

In conclusion, progressing your chair yoga practice to intermediate poses is a natural evolution that brings a wealth of benefits, including increased strength, flexibility, and heightened mind-body awareness. This comprehensive guide serves as a valuable resource for individuals seeking to elevate their chair yoga experience. By understanding the significance of progression, exploring the benefits of intermediate poses, and incorporating practical tips into your practice, you can embark on a transformative journey that nurtures both your physical and mental well-being. Remember to approach your practice with patience, mindfulness, and a sense of curiosity as you explore the enriching world of intermediate chair yoga poses.

CHAPTER 16: CHAIR YOGA SEQUENCES FOR MORNING AND EVENING ROUTINES

Yoga, a practice deeply rooted in mindfulness and holistic well-being, extends its transformative benefits to chair yoga, making it accessible to individuals of all ages and abilities. This comprehensive guide explores the art of crafting chair yoga sequences specifically tailored for morning and evening routines. From invigorating poses to start the day with vitality to calming stretches to wind down in the evening, this guide delves into the significance of incorporating chair yoga into your daily regimen and provides detailed sequences to optimize both the beginning and the end of your day.

Morning Chair Yoga Sequence: Awakening Vitality

1. **Seated Neck Stretches:**

   - Sit tall in the chair, gently tilt the head to one side, feeling a stretch along the neck.

   - Repeat on the other side and incorporate gentle neck circles.

   - Benefits: Relieves tension, improves neck flexibility, and enhances blood circulation to the brain.

2. **Chair Cat-Cow Stretch:**

   - Sit at the edge of the chair with hands on knees.

   - Inhale, arch the back, and lift the chest (Cow).

   - Exhale, round the spine, and tuck the chin to the chest (Cat).

   - Benefits: Warms up the spine, massages internal organs,

and promotes flexibility.

3. **Seated Sun Salutations:**
   - Inhale, reach the arms overhead, and interlace the fingers.
   - Exhale, lean to one side, stretching the side body.
   - Inhale back to center and repeat on the other side.
   - Benefits: Energizes the entire body, improves circulation, and enhances flexibility.

4. **Seated Forward Fold:**
   - Sit tall with legs extended.
   - Hinge at the hips, bringing the chest forward and reaching towards the toes.
   - Hold for a few breaths, feeling the stretch in the hamstrings and lower back.
   - Benefits: Stimulates digestion, stretches the spine, and awakens the back body.

5. **Chair Mountain Pose:**
   - Sit with feet hip-width apart, grounding through the sit bones.
   - Inhale, reach the arms overhead, palms facing each other.
   - Engage the core and lift through the chest.
   - Benefits: Builds strength in the core, improves posture, and invigorates the entire body.

6. **Seated Twist with Arm Reach:**
   - Sit tall and twist gently, bringing one hand to the opposite knee.
   - Inhale, reach the opposite arm overhead.
   - Hold for a few breaths, engaging the core.

- Benefits: Stimulates digestion, improves spinal mobility, and stretches the torso.

7. **Chair Warrior II:**
    - Sit at the edge of the chair, extend one leg forward, and bend the other knee.
    - Arms parallel to the ground, gaze over the front fingertips.
    - Hold the pose, engaging the core and grounding through the sit bones.
    - Benefits: Strengthens the legs, opens the hips, and builds focus.

8. **Chair Tree Pose:**
    - Sit tall with feet flat on the floor.
    - Lift one foot and place it on the inner calf or ankle.
    - Hold the pose, finding a focal point for balance.
    - Benefits: Enhances balance, strengthens the legs, and promotes concentration.

9. **Chair Forward Fold with Arm Extension:**
    - Sit tall and hinge at the hips, reaching the arms forward.
    - Hold the pose, feeling a stretch in the spine and shoulders.
    - Benefits: Lengthens the spine, stretches the shoulders, and encourages a sense of grounding.

10. **Final Relaxation:**
    - End the morning sequence with a few minutes of seated meditation or deep breathing.
    - Reflect on intentions for the day ahead.

Evening Chair Yoga Sequence: Unwinding Tranquility

1. **Gentle Seated Side Bends:**

- Inhale, lift one arm overhead, and gently bend to the side.
- Feel the stretch along the side of the body.
- Hold, then return to the center and repeat on the other side.
- Benefits: Relaxes the side body, opens the intercostal muscles, and promotes gentle stretching.

2. **Seated Spinal Twist:**

- Sit tall and twist gently, bringing the opposite hand to the outer knee.
- Observe the twist in the spine and the breath.
- Repeat on the other side.
- Benefits: Releases tension in the spine, massages abdominal organs, and calms the nervous system.

3. **Seated Wide-Legged Forward Fold:**

- Sit with legs extended wide apart.
- Hinge forward from the hips, maintaining a straight spine.
- Mindfully explore the stretch along the inner thighs and spine.
- Benefits: Stretches the inner thighs, releases tension in the lower back, and promotes relaxation.

4. **Chair Child's Pose:**

- Sit back in the chair, reaching the arms forward.
- Allow the chest to rest on the thighs and the forehead on the arms.
- Benefits: Stretches the back, shoulders, and promotes a sense of surrender.

5. **Seated Eagle Arms:**

- Sit tall, extend the arms forward, and cross one arm over the other, wrapping them around each other.
- Lift the elbows and drop the shoulders, feeling a stretch in the upper back.
- Benefits: Relieves tension in the shoulders, opens the upper back, and encourages deep breathing.

6. Chair Pigeon Pose:

- Sit on the edge of the chair, cross one ankle over the opposite knee.
- Gently lean forward, keeping the back straight.
- Benefits: Stretches the hips, releases tension in the glutes, and promotes relaxation.

7. Seated Butterfly Stretch:

- Sit tall, bring the soles of the feet together, and gently press the knees toward the floor.
- Hold the pose, feeling a stretch in the inner thighs.
- Benefits: Opens the hips, releases tension in the groin, and encourages relaxation.

8. Seated Supported Heart Opener:

- Place a cushion or bolster behind the lower back while seated.
- Lean back against the support, allowing the chest to open.
- Benefits: Releases tension in the chest, stretches the front body, and promotes a sense of calm.

9. Chair Legs Up the Wall Variation:

- Sit sideways in the chair and extend the legs up the wall, if available.
- Allow the arms to rest by the sides.
- Benefits: Promotes circulation, relieves swelling in the

legs, and induces a calming effect.

10. **Guided Relaxation or Meditation:**

- Conclude the evening sequence with a guided relaxation or meditation.
- Focus on calming breathwork and releasing any remaining tension.

Tips for Optimizing Chair Yoga Routines:

- **Adapt Poses to Your Comfort:**
  - Modify poses based on your comfort level and any physical considerations.
  - Chair yoga is versatile, and poses can be adapted to suit individual needs.

- **Mindful Breathing:**
  - Incorporate mindful breathing throughout the sequences.
  - Focus on deep inhales and exhales to enhance the mind-body connection.

- **Integrate Props:**
  - Use props such as cushions, blankets, or yoga blocks to enhance comfort and support.
  - Props can assist in achieving proper alignment and relaxation.

- **Set Intentions:**
  - Begin each sequence with a mindful intention for the practice.
  - Setting intentions creates a sense of purpose and mindfulness.

- **Listen to Your Body:**
  - Pay attention to how your body responds to each pose.
  - If a pose causes discomfort, ease into it

gradually or skip it altogether.

- **Consistency is Key:**
    - Establish a consistent routine for morning and evening chair yoga.
    - Regular practice enhances the cumulative benefits of the sequences.

- **Create a Relaxing Environment:**
    - Choose a quiet and comfortable space for your chair yoga practice.
    - Dim the lights in the evening to promote a calming atmosphere.

- **Stay Present:**
    - Throughout the sequences, stay present and fully engaged in each movement.
    - Mindful presence amplifies the therapeutic effects of chair yoga.

Conclusion:

In conclusion, chair yoga sequences designed for morning and evening routines offer a harmonious blend of energizing and calming poses, catering to the specific needs of each part of the day. Whether you seek to invigorate your morning with vitality or wind down in the evening for a restful night's sleep, chair yoga provides a versatile and accessible practice. This comprehensive guide serves as a valuable resource for individuals looking to integrate chair yoga into their daily regimen, fostering a balanced and mindful approach to well-being. Embrace the transformative power of chair yoga as you embark on a journey of self-care and holistic health, creating a foundation for vitality in the morning and tranquility in the evening.

CHAPTER 17: INCORPORATING PROPS FOR ADDED COMFORT AND SUPPORT

Chair yoga, with its gentle and accessible nature, becomes even more enriching when enhanced by the thoughtful integration of props. Props play a pivotal role in chair yoga, offering added comfort, support, and accessibility to individuals of varying abilities and physical conditions. This comprehensive guide delves into the significance of incorporating props into chair yoga practices, the benefits they provide, and a detailed exploration of how different props can be utilized to enhance comfort and support.

Significance of Props in Chair Yoga:

- **Enhanced Comfort:**
    - Props, such as cushions, blankets, or bolsters, are instrumental in providing additional padding and support, ensuring that individuals experience maximum comfort during their practice.
    - Enhanced comfort allows for a more enjoyable and sustainable yoga experience.

- **Improved Alignment:**
    - Props assist in achieving optimal alignment in various poses, helping individuals maintain proper posture and reduce the risk of strain or discomfort.
    - Proper alignment contributes to the effectiveness of each pose and promotes overall safety.

- **Accessibility for All:**
    - Props make chair yoga accessible to a diverse range of practitioners, including those with limited mobility, injuries, or chronic conditions.
    - With the right use of props, individuals of all ages and physical abilities can engage in a supportive yoga practice.

- **Deepening Stretches:**
    - Utilizing props allows individuals to deepen stretches safely, gradually increasing flexibility without compromising stability.
    - Props offer a controlled and supportive environment for practitioners to explore their range of motion.

- **Mind-Body Connection:**
    - Props encourage a deeper mind-body connection by promoting relaxation and reducing unnecessary physical strain.
    - With the aid of props, individuals can focus more on breath, mindfulness, and the overall experience of their practice.

Types of Props in Chair Yoga:

- **Cushions and Pillows:**
    - Placing cushions or pillows under the seat or behind the back provides additional support and comfort.
    - Cushions can be used to modify seated poses, making them more accessible and enjoyable.

- **Blankets:**
    - Blankets can be folded or rolled to support different parts of the body, such as the knees, lower back, or neck.

- They add a layer of comfort during relaxation poses and help maintain warmth during the practice.

- **Bolsters:**
  - Bolsters offer support for various poses, particularly those involving forward folds or gentle backbends.
  - Placing a bolster under the knees or lower back enhances relaxation and reduces strain.

- **Yoga Blocks:**
  - Yoga blocks can be used to modify the height or distance of certain poses, ensuring proper alignment.
  - They are particularly helpful for individuals who may need additional lift or support in seated or standing poses.

- **Straps:**
  - Straps assist in achieving a comfortable reach in poses that involve holding onto the feet or legs.
  - They are beneficial for individuals with limited flexibility, allowing them to gradually improve their range of motion.

- **Resistance Bands:**
  - Resistance bands add an element of gentle strength training to chair yoga.
  - They can be incorporated to enhance the engagement of muscles in various poses, promoting stability and strength.

- **Chair:**
  - The chair itself is a fundamental prop in chair yoga.

- It provides stability, support, and serves as a versatile tool for seated poses, standing poses, and modifications.

How to Incorporate Props into Chair Yoga:

1. Seated Meditation with Cushion:

- Place a cushion under the seat to elevate the hips and provide a comfortable foundation for seated meditation.
- This promotes proper alignment, reduces pressure on the lower back, and encourages a relaxed posture.

2. Supported Forward Fold with Blanket:

- Sit at the edge of the chair and drape a folded blanket over the thighs.
- Hinge forward at the hips, allowing the blanket to support the upper body weight.
- This modification enhances the stretch in the lower back and hamstrings.

3. Chair Supported Warrior II with Blocks:

- Use yoga blocks to modify Warrior II by placing them under the front foot for added height.
- This modification supports stability, making the pose more accessible and comfortable.

4. Gentle Backbend with Bolster:

- Sit at the edge of the chair, placing a bolster behind the lower back.
- Lean back gently, allowing the bolster to support the spine in a mild backbend.
- This modification encourages a gentle opening of the chest and heart center.

5. Chair Supported Tree Pose with Chair:

- Hold onto the back of the chair for support while

practicing Tree Pose.

- The chair provides stability, allowing practitioners to focus on balance and alignment without the fear of falling.

6. Seated Twist with Strap:

- Sit tall, extend one leg, and loop a strap around the foot.
- Gently twist towards the extended leg, using the strap to support the movement.
- This modification enhances the stretch in the spine and shoulders.

7. Chair Supported Hip Opener with Blocks:

- Place yoga blocks under the knees while seated to support and elevate the legs.
- This modification creates a comfortable hip-opening stretch and reduces strain on the lower back.

8. Chair-Assisted Downward-Facing Dog:

- Stand facing the chair, placing hands on the seat.
- Walk the feet back to create a downward-facing dog shape.
- The chair provides stability and support, making the pose accessible.

Tips for Effective Use of Props:

- **Understand Individual Needs:**
  - Assess the unique needs of practitioners and choose props accordingly.
  - Understanding individual requirements ensures that props serve their intended purpose.
- **Provide Options:**
  - Offer variations with and without props

to accommodate different preferences and comfort levels.

- Providing options allows practitioners to choose the level of support they need.

- **Educate Practitioners:**
  - Educate practitioners on the proper use of props and their benefits.
  - Encourage self-exploration and adjustments to find the most comfortable variations.

- **Regular Prop Maintenance:**
  - Ensure that props are in good condition, free from wear and tear.
  - Regular maintenance guarantees the safety and effectiveness of props during practice.

- **Experiment with Different Props:**
  - Experiment with various props to discover the combination that works best for each individual.
  - Some practitioners may prefer a combination of props for optimal comfort.

- **Encourage Prop Modifications:**
  - Encourage practitioners to modify or adjust props as needed.
  - Modification promotes a sense of empowerment and allows individuals to tailor their practice.

- **Be Mindful of Accessibility:**
  - Ensure that props are easily accessible for all practitioners.
  - Consider the placement of props to minimize disruptions during the practice.

- **Incorporate Props Gradually:**

- ◦ Introduce props gradually, allowing practitioners to acclimate to their use.
- ◦ Gradual incorporation ensures a smooth transition and enhances the overall experience.

Conclusion:

In conclusion, the thoughtful incorporation of props into chair yoga practices elevates the experience, making it more inclusive, comfortable, and supportive for individuals of all abilities. This comprehensive guide serves as a valuable resource for understanding the significance of props in chair yoga, the types of props available, and practical ways to integrate them into various poses. By embracing the versatility and benefits of props, practitioners can cultivate a personalized and enriching chair yoga practice that nurtures both the body and the mind. Props become allies in the journey of well-being, providing a foundation for comfort, support, and the exploration of yoga's transformative potential within the accessible realm of chair yoga.

CHAPTER 18: CHAIR YOGA FOR BETTER SLEEP AND RELAXATION

As our lives become increasingly hectic and stress-laden, the quest for better sleep and relaxation has become more crucial than ever. In this pursuit, chair yoga emerges as a gentle yet powerful practice that offers a therapeutic approach to achieving restful nights and deep relaxation. This comprehensive guide explores the significance of chair yoga in promoting better sleep, delving into the science behind its efficacy, the specific poses tailored for relaxation, and practical tips for incorporating this practice into your bedtime routine.

Understanding the Connection Between Chair Yoga and Sleep:

- **Stress Reduction:**
    - Chair yoga integrates gentle movements, breathwork, and mindfulness, creating a holistic approach to stress reduction.
    - By alleviating stress, the practice prepares the body and mind for a more peaceful transition into sleep.

- **Cortisol Regulation:**
    - The controlled and intentional movements in chair yoga contribute to the regulation of cortisol, the stress hormone.
    - Balancing cortisol levels helps create an optimal environment for the body to unwind and embrace rest.

- **Mind-Body Connection:**
    - Chair yoga fosters a deep mind-body

connection, encouraging individuals to be present and attentive to their physical sensations.

- This heightened awareness facilitates the release of tension and promotes a sense of relaxation.

- **Calming the Nervous System:**
  - The gentle stretches and breath-focused practices in chair yoga activate the parasympathetic nervous system.
  - Activating the "rest and digest" mode counteracts the effects of the sympathetic nervous system, inducing a state of calmness.

Chair Yoga Poses for Better Sleep:

- **Seated Cat-Cow Stretch:**
  - Sit at the edge of the chair and flow between arching and rounding the spine.
  - This gentle movement releases tension in the back and promotes a sense of ease.

- **Forward Fold with Support:**
  - Hinge forward from the hips while seated, supporting the forehead with folded arms or a cushion.
  - This pose elongates the spine, relaxes the neck, and calms the mind.

- **Supported Child's Pose:**
  - Sit back on the chair, reaching the arms forward and resting the chest on the thighs.
  - This restorative pose provides a sense of surrender, releasing tension from the back and shoulders.

- **Seated Twist with Gentle Neck Stretch:**

- Gently twist the torso while seated and add a gentle neck stretch by tilting the head to one side.
- This combination relieves tension in the spine and neck, promoting relaxation.

- **Legs Up the Chair Pose:**
  - Lie on your back with the legs resting on the seat of a chair.
  - This inversion promotes blood circulation, reduces swelling in the legs, and induces a calming effect.

- **Seated Meditation with Deep Breathing:**
  - Sit comfortably in the chair, close your eyes, and focus on deep, rhythmic breathing.
  - Mindful breathing activates the relaxation response, preparing the body for sleep.

- **Gentle Shoulder Rolls:**
  - Sit tall and roll the shoulders in gentle, circular motions.
  - This simple movement releases tension in the shoulders and upper back.

- **Chair Supported Savasana:**
  - Lie back on the chair with legs extended and arms resting by your sides.
  - This supported relaxation pose allows for complete surrender and tranquility.

Practical Tips for Incorporating Chair Yoga into Your Bedtime Routine:

- **Create a Calming Environment:**
  - Set up a serene space for your chair yoga practice with dim lighting and soothing elements.

- Creating a calming environment enhances the effectiveness of the practice.

- **Establish a Consistent Routine:**
  - Incorporate chair yoga into your bedtime routine consistently.
  - A regular practice signals to the body that it's time to wind down and prepare for sleep.

- **Mindful Transition from Day to Night:**
  - Use chair yoga as a mindful transition from the activities of the day to the stillness of the night.
  - This intentional shift primes the body and mind for rest.

- **Focus on Breath Awareness:**
  - Emphasize mindful breathing throughout your chair yoga practice.
  - Conscious breathing activates the relaxation response, promoting a tranquil state.

- **Progressive Relaxation Techniques:**
  - Incorporate progressive relaxation by consciously relaxing each part of the body during your practice.
  - This technique promotes a profound sense of ease and relaxation.

- **Limit Stimulants Before Bed:**
  - Avoid stimulating activities, caffeine, or heavy meals close to bedtime.
  - Opt for chair yoga as a gentle and calming alternative to winding down.

- **Use Comfortable Props:**
  - Enhance your comfort with supportive props like cushions or blankets.
  - Comfortable props create a nurturing

environment for relaxation.

- **Mindful Transitions Between Poses:**
  - Transition between chair yoga poses mindfully and with awareness.
  - Slow and intentional movements prepare the body for a serene and restful state.

Scientific Insights into Chair Yoga and Sleep:

- **Neurotransmitter Regulation:**
  - Chair yoga has been associated with the regulation of neurotransmitters, such as serotonin and melatonin, which play a crucial role in sleep-wake cycles.
  - Enhanced regulation contributes to improved sleep quality.

- **Heart Rate Variability (HRV):**
  - Research suggests that chair yoga positively influences heart rate variability, an indicator of the body's ability to adapt to stress.
  - Improved HRV is linked to better sleep patterns.

- **Circadian Rhythm Alignment:**
  - Consistent chair yoga practice may contribute to the alignment of the circadian rhythm.
  - A balanced circadian rhythm supports the natural sleep-wake cycle.

- **Reduced Insomnia Symptoms:**
  - Studies have indicated that regular chair yoga practice is associated with a reduction in symptoms of insomnia.
  - Individuals report falling asleep faster and experiencing deeper sleep.

Conclusion:

In conclusion, chair yoga stands as a beacon of solace for those seeking better sleep and profound relaxation. This comprehensive guide has explored the synergistic relationship between chair yoga and improved sleep, the specific poses tailored for relaxation, and practical tips for seamlessly incorporating this practice into your bedtime routine. The gentle nature of chair yoga, coupled with its mindful and intentional approach, provides a therapeutic pathway to unwind the body and calm the mind. By embracing chair yoga as a bedtime ritual, individuals can foster a deep connection with their well-being, facilitating restful nights and awakening rejuvenated to the possibilities of a new day. Embrace the transformative power of chair yoga as you embark on a journey towards enhanced sleep and profound relaxation, finding sanctuary in the gentle embrace of this accessible and therapeutic practice.

CHAPTER 19: UNDERSTANDING THE MIND-BODY CONNECTION IN CHAIR YOGA

Chair yoga, a gentle and accessible form of yoga, places a profound emphasis on the mind-body connection. This comprehensive guide delves into the intricate relationship between the mind and body within the context of chair yoga. By understanding this connection, practitioners can harness the therapeutic benefits of the practice, promoting holistic well-being, and cultivating a harmonious equilibrium between mental and physical health.

Foundations of the Mind-Body Connection in Chair Yoga:

- **Holistic Approach:**
    - Chair yoga, rooted in the ancient principles of yoga, embraces a holistic approach to well-being.
    - It recognizes that the mind and body are interconnected, and the health of one significantly influences the other.

- **Conscious Breathwork:**
    - Central to chair yoga is the practice of conscious breathwork, or pranayama.
    - Mindful breathing serves as a bridge between the mental and physical realms, fostering awareness and relaxation.

- **Intentional Movement:**
    - The intentional and mindful movements in chair yoga serve as a vehicle for cultivating awareness.

- Each movement becomes an opportunity to unite the mind and body in a harmonious dance of presence and consciousness.

- **Focused Awareness:**
  - Chair yoga encourages practitioners to bring focused awareness to the sensations, thoughts, and emotions arising during the practice.
  - This heightened awareness deepens the mind-body connection, fostering a sense of unity.

The Science Behind Mind-Body Connection in Chair Yoga:

- **Neurotransmitter Release:**
  - Mindful movements and breathwork in chair yoga stimulate the release of neurotransmitters like serotonin and dopamine.
  - These neurotransmitters contribute to mood regulation, creating a positive impact on mental well-being.

- **Stress Response Reduction:**
  - The mind-body connection in chair yoga activates the parasympathetic nervous system, reducing the stress response.
  - This shift from the "fight or flight" response to the "rest and digest" mode promotes relaxation and mental calmness.

- **Cortisol Regulation:**
  - Mindful chair yoga practices contribute to the regulation of cortisol, the stress hormone.
  - Balancing cortisol levels is crucial for reducing stress, anxiety, and promoting a sense of tranquility.

- **Enhanced Brain Function:**
  - Studies suggest that regular yoga practices,

including chair yoga, positively impact brain function.

- ◦ Improved cognitive function, memory, and attention are linked to the mind-body connection cultivated in yoga.

Components of Mind-Body Connection in Chair Yoga:

- **Breath-Aware Movement:**
    - ◦ The essence of chair yoga lies in synchronized breath-aware movement.
    - ◦ Practitioners consciously link each breath with movement, fostering a deep connection between the breath, body, and mind.

- **Body Scan and Awareness:**
    - ◦ Chair yoga often incorporates body scan techniques, where practitioners mindfully explore and bring awareness to different parts of the body.
    - ◦ This practice deepens the connection between mental awareness and physical sensations.

- **Meditative Practices:**
    - ◦ Meditation, an integral part of chair yoga, deepens the mind-body connection by encouraging inner stillness and heightened awareness.
    - ◦ Practices such as mindful breathing or guided meditation foster mental clarity and tranquility.

- **Visualization Techniques:**
    - ◦ Chair yoga frequently integrates visualization techniques where practitioners focus their mind on positive imagery.
    - ◦ Visualization enhances the mind-body

connection by engaging the imagination and emotions.

- **Affirmations and Positive Intentions:**
    - Affirmations and setting positive intentions during chair yoga reinforce a positive mindset.
    - The repetition of affirmations creates a powerful mental environment that influences physical well-being.

Mind-Body Connection in Specific Chair Yoga Poses:

- **Seated Mountain Pose:**
    - Sitting tall with feet grounded, this pose encourages an awareness of posture and a sense of groundedness.
    - Practitioners connect with their breath, fostering mental focus and stability.

- **Chair Cat-Cow Stretch:**
    - Flowing between arching and rounding the spine while seated promotes a conscious connection with breath and movement.
    - This dynamic stretch enhances the mind-body link by encouraging fluidity and awareness.

- **Seated Forward Fold:**
    - Hinging forward from the hips while seated directs attention to the sensations in the hamstrings and lower back.
    - The stretch promotes introspection and mindful release of tension.

- **Gentle Seated Twist:**
    - Twisting gently while seated encourages the release of tension in the spine and enhances spinal flexibility.
    - Practitioners connect with their breath and the

subtle sensations in the body.

- **Chair Warrior Pose:**
    - This modified version of the traditional Warrior Pose encourages strength, stability, and focused attention.
    - The mind engages with the body's strength and balance in this empowering posture.

- **Chair Tree Pose:**
    - Balancing on one leg while seated in a chair fosters concentration, balance, and a deep sense of presence.
    - Practitioners connect with the sensations of grounding and stability.

- **Chair Savasana:**
    - The classic relaxation pose in a seated position, Chair Savasana, promotes deep rest and introspection.
    - Practitioners cultivate awareness of breath, sensations, and the profound relaxation of the body and mind.

Practical Tips for Deepening the Mind-Body Connection in Chair Yoga:

- **Set an Intention:**
    - Begin each chair yoga session with a mindful intention.
    - Setting an intention anchors the practice in purpose and mindfulness.

- **Cultivate Breath Awareness:**
    - Emphasize conscious and deep breathing throughout the practice.
    - Breath awareness serves as a constant thread connecting the mind and body.

- **Practice Mindful Transitions:**
    - Transition between chair yoga poses mindfully, maintaining awareness of each movement.
    - Mindful transitions deepen the connection between mental focus and physical engagement.
- **Explore Sensations:**
    - Encourage practitioners to explore sensations within each pose.
    - The mindful exploration of physical sensations deepens the mind-body connection.
- **Use Guided Imagery:**
    - Integrate guided imagery or visualization techniques during chair yoga sessions.
    - Visualization engages the mind, fostering a deeper connection with the body.
- **Incorporate Affirmations:**
    - Introduce positive affirmations during chair yoga to enhance the mental and emotional aspects of the practice.
    - Affirmations contribute to a positive mind-body connection.
- **Encourage Self-Reflection:**
    - Conclude chair yoga sessions with a moment of self-reflection.
    - Encouraging practitioners to reflect on their experience deepens the understanding of the mind-body connection.
- **Practice Regularly:**
    - Consistent chair yoga practice is key to deepening the mind-body connection.
    - Regular practice establishes a routine that

reinforces the integration of mental and physical well-being.

Realizing the Benefits of a Strong Mind-Body Connection:

- **Stress Reduction:**
    - A strong mind-body connection established through chair yoga contributes to stress reduction.
    - Mindful awareness mitigates the impact of stressors on both mental and physical well-being.

- **Enhanced Emotional Well-Being:**
    - The mind-body connection nurtured in chair yoga positively influences emotional well-being.
    - Practitioners develop resilience and emotional awareness through the practice.

- **Improved Physical Health:**
    - As mental well-being improves, physical health follows suit.
    - Reduced stress and enhanced relaxation contribute to overall physical health and vitality.

- **Greater Mindfulness in Daily Life:**
    - The mindfulness cultivated in chair yoga extends into daily life.
    - Practitioners carry the benefits of a strong mind-body connection into their interactions, decision-making, and overall lifestyle.

- **Optimized Cognitive Function:**
    - The holistic benefits of chair yoga, including improved cognitive function, positively impact mental clarity and focus.

- Enhanced cognitive function supports overall mental acuity.

Scientific Perspectives on Mind-Body Connection in Yoga:

- **Psychoneuroimmunology:**
    - The field of psychoneuroimmunology explores the interconnectedness of the mind, nervous system, and immune system.
    - Chair yoga's impact on stress reduction may contribute to improved immune function.

- **Mindfulness-Based Stress Reduction (MBSR):**
    - Mindfulness-based practices, including chair yoga, are associated with the Mindfulness-Based Stress Reduction (MBSR) approach.
    - MBSR has shown efficacy in promoting mental well-being and reducing stress.

- **Neuroplasticity:**
    - Research on neuroplasticity suggests that the brain has the ability to adapt and rewire.
    - Consistent chair yoga practice may contribute to positive changes in neural pathways, influencing mental health.

- **Heart-Brain Connection:**
    - The heart and brain are intricately connected through the autonomic nervous system.
    - Mind-body practices like chair yoga positively influence heart rate variability, promoting cardiovascular health and mental well-being.

Conclusion:

In conclusion, chair yoga serves as a gateway to understanding and harnessing the intricate mind-body connection. This comprehensive guide has explored the foundational principles, scientific underpinnings, specific chair yoga poses, and practical tips for deepening the mind-body connection. The practice of chair yoga offers a sanctuary where practitioners can cultivate awareness, balance, and integration between the mental and physical realms. By embracing the transformative potential of the mind-body connection in chair yoga, individuals embark on a journey toward holistic well-being, fostering resilience, tranquility, and a profound sense of self-awareness. As the mind and body dance in harmony through the art of chair yoga, practitioners unlock a path to inner peace, vitality, and a richer, more meaningful life.

CHAPTER 20: NUTRITION TIPS TO ENHANCE THE BENEFITS OF CHAIR YOGA

The synergistic relationship between nutrition and chair yoga forms a powerful foundation for holistic well-being. This comprehensive guide explores the intricate connection between what we eat and the benefits derived from chair yoga. By integrating mindful nutrition practices with chair yoga, practitioners can enhance physical vitality, mental clarity, and overall health. This detailed exploration delves into the principles of mindful eating, nutritional considerations for chair yoga practitioners, and practical tips for optimizing the benefits of both practices.

Principles of Mindful Nutrition:

- **Conscious Eating:**
    - Mindful nutrition begins with conscious eating, where individuals savor each bite with awareness.
    - Chair yoga practitioners can apply mindfulness to their meals, fostering a deeper connection with the nourishment they provide.

- **Balanced Nutrition:**
    - Ensure a well-balanced diet that includes a variety of nutrients.
    - A balance of carbohydrates, proteins, healthy fats, vitamins, and minerals supports the body's energy levels and overall functioning.

- **Hydration:**
    - Proper hydration is crucial for optimal bodily

functions.

- Drinking an adequate amount of water supports joint flexibility, digestion, and overall vitality—complementing the benefits of chair yoga.

- **Whole Foods Emphasis:**
    - Prioritize whole, unprocessed foods rich in nutrients.
    - Whole foods provide essential vitamins and minerals that contribute to overall health, aligning with the holistic principles of chair yoga.

Nutritional Considerations for Chair Yoga Practitioners:

- **Pre-Practice Nutrition:**
    - Consume a balanced meal containing complex carbohydrates, lean proteins, and healthy fats before chair yoga.
    - Pre-practice nutrition provides sustained energy, enhancing the practitioner's ability to engage in the practice with focus and vitality.

- **Post-Practice Nutrition:**
    - After chair yoga, prioritize a nutritious post-practice meal or snack.
    - Nutrient-dense foods replenish energy stores and support muscle recovery, optimizing the benefits gained from the practice.

- **Protein Intake:**
    - Incorporate adequate protein into the diet to support muscle maintenance and recovery.
    - Protein-rich foods like lean meats, legumes, and dairy contribute to overall strength and flexibility, key elements in chair yoga.

- **Anti-Inflammatory Foods:**
  - Include anti-inflammatory foods such as fruits, vegetables, fatty fish, and nuts in the diet.
  - These foods help manage inflammation, supporting joint health and flexibility—a crucial aspect of chair yoga.

- **Balancing Blood Sugar Levels:**
  - Consume complex carbohydrates, fiber-rich foods, and healthy fats to balance blood sugar levels.
  - Stable blood sugar levels promote sustained energy during chair yoga sessions.

- **Mindful Eating Practices:**
  - Practice mindful eating by savoring each bite, chewing slowly, and paying attention to hunger and fullness cues.
  - Mindful eating fosters a deeper connection with food, promoting a holistic approach to nutrition.

- **Hydration Strategies:**
  - Stay well-hydrated throughout the day, particularly before and after chair yoga sessions.
  - Hydration supports joint lubrication, flexibility, and overall well-being.

Nutrition Tips for Enhanced Chair Yoga Benefits:

- **Pre-Practice Snack Ideas:**
  - Choose a pre-practice snack with a mix of carbohydrates and protein.
  - Options include a banana with nut butter, yogurt with granola, or a small smoothie with fruits and greens.

- **Post-Practice Meal Options:**
    - Opt for a balanced post-practice meal containing lean protein, whole grains, and plenty of vegetables.
    - Grilled chicken with quinoa and a colorful vegetable medley is an example of a nourishing post-practice meal.
- **Herbal Teas for Relaxation:**
    - Incorporate calming herbal teas like chamomile or peppermint after evening chair yoga sessions.
    - Herbal teas contribute to relaxation, aligning with the calming effects of chair yoga.
- **Omega-3 Fatty Acids for Joint Health:**
    - Include sources of omega-3 fatty acids such as fatty fish, flaxseeds, and walnuts in the diet.
    - Omega-3s support joint health, enhancing the benefits of chair yoga for flexibility.
- **Colorful Plate Approach:**
    - Aim for a colorful plate with a variety of fruits and vegetables.
    - Different colors indicate diverse nutrients, promoting overall health and vitality.
- **Mindful Snacking:**
    - Choose mindful snacks like a handful of nuts, yogurt with berries, or sliced veggies with hummus.
    - Mindful snacking provides sustained energy between chair yoga sessions.
- **Probiotics for Digestive Health:**
    - Incorporate probiotic-rich foods like yogurt, kefir, and sauerkraut for digestive health.

- - A healthy digestive system complements the holistic benefits of chair yoga.
- **Homemade Energy Bites:**
  - Prepare homemade energy bites with ingredients like oats, nuts, seeds, and dried fruits.
  - These bites serve as convenient and nourishing snacks for sustained energy.

Meal Timing and Chair Yoga Practice:

- **Pre-Practice Meal Timing:**
  - Consume a balanced meal containing carbohydrates and proteins 1-2 hours before chair yoga.
  - This timing allows for proper digestion and energy release during the practice.
- **Post-Practice Meal Timing:**
  - Aim to eat a nutrient-dense post-practice meal within 1-2 hours after chair yoga.
  - This window supports muscle recovery and replenishes energy stores.
- **Hydration Timing:**
  - Stay hydrated throughout the day and prioritize hydration before and after chair yoga.
  - Adequate hydration supports joint flexibility and overall well-being.

Nutrition for Stress Management:

- **Adaptogenic Herbs:**
  - Consider incorporating adaptogenic herbs like ashwagandha or tulsi into the diet.
  - These herbs support the body's ability to manage stress, complementing the stress-reducing benefits of chair yoga.

- **Complex Carbohydrates for Serotonin Production:**
    - Include complex carbohydrates like whole grains and legumes.
    - Complex carbohydrates contribute to serotonin production, promoting a sense of calmness and well-being.
- **Magnesium-Rich Foods:**
    - Consume magnesium-rich foods such as leafy greens, nuts, and seeds.
    - Magnesium supports relaxation and may alleviate muscle tension—an excellent complement to chair yoga practice.

Scientific Insights into Nutrition and Yoga:

- **Gut-Brain Axis:**
    - Research on the gut-brain axis highlights the interconnectedness of gut health and mental well-being.
    - A well-balanced diet supports gut health, influencing mood and cognitive function—a key consideration in chair yoga practice.
- **Nutrient-Dense Diet and Cognitive Function:**
    - Studies suggest that a nutrient-dense diet positively impacts cognitive function.
    - Enhanced cognitive function supports mental clarity, focus, and mindfulness—a synergy with chair yoga.
- **Inflammation and Joint Health:**
    - Nutritional choices play a role in managing inflammation, affecting joint health.
    - Anti-inflammatory foods contribute to the joint-supportive benefits of chair yoga.
- **Hydration and Physical Performance:**

- ◦ Proper hydration is essential for physical performance and flexibility.
- ◦ Hydration supports joint lubrication, aiding in the fluid movements of chair yoga poses.

Conclusion:

In conclusion, the fusion of mindful nutrition with chair yoga creates a harmonious path to holistic well-being. This comprehensive guide has explored the principles of mindful nutrition, nutritional considerations for chair yoga practitioners, and practical tips for optimizing the benefits of both practices. By approaching nutrition with intention and mindfulness, individuals can enhance the physical and mental benefits derived from chair yoga. As chair yoga nourishes the body and mind, thoughtful nutrition becomes the fuel that sustains and amplifies these transformative effects. Embrace the synergy of mindful nutrition and chair yoga, cultivating a holistic approach to well-being that radiates from the inside out—a journey toward vitality, balance, and lasting health.

CHAPTER 21: THE 21-DAY CHAIR YOGA CHALLENGE: DAILY PRACTICES FOR WEIGHT LOSS AND OVERALL WELL-BEING

Embarking on a transformative journey, the 21-Day Chair Yoga Challenge intertwines the principles of yoga, the accessibility of chair-based exercises, and a commitment to daily practice. Designed to foster weight loss and enhance overall well-being, this challenge combines mindful movement, breathwork, and self-care. This comprehensive guide delves into the intricacies of the 21-Day Chair Yoga Challenge, exploring the daily practices, the holistic approach to weight loss, and the profound impact on physical and mental well-being.

Foundation of the 21-Day Chair Yoga Challenge:

- **Commitment to Consistency:**
    - The challenge emphasizes daily engagement in chair yoga practices for 21 days.
    - Consistent practice fosters habit formation, allowing participants to experience the cumulative benefits of chair yoga.

- **Accessible Yoga for All Ages:**
    - Chair yoga ensures accessibility for individuals of all ages and fitness levels.
    - This inclusivity makes the challenge suitable for beginners and those seeking a gentle yet effective approach to weight loss.

- **Mindful Integration of Yoga Principles:**
    - The challenge incorporates key yoga principles

such as breath awareness, mindfulness, and holistic well-being.

- These principles create a foundation for self-discovery, promoting a balanced approach to weight loss.

Daily Practices of the 21-Day Chair Yoga Challenge:

- **Day 1-5: Foundations of Chair Yoga:**
    - Establish foundational postures and breathwork techniques.
    - Focus on building awareness of body alignment and breath, laying the groundwork for the subsequent practices.

- **Day 6-10: Energizing Chair Yoga Flows:**
    - Introduce dynamic chair yoga flows to increase energy and circulation.
    - These sequences aim to elevate heart rate gently, contributing to calorie expenditure and boosting metabolism.

- **Day 11-15: Core-Strengthening Chair Yoga Poses:**
    - Emphasize core-strengthening postures to engage abdominal muscles.
    - Strengthening the core not only supports weight loss but also enhances overall stability and posture.

- **Day 16-20: Chair Yoga for Flexibility:**
    - Integrate stretches and flexibility-focused poses.
    - Improved flexibility aids in increased range of motion, reduces stiffness, and complements weight loss efforts.

- **Day 21: Culmination and Reflection:**
    - Conclude the challenge with a comprehensive

chair yoga session.

- ◦ Encourage participants to reflect on their journey, celebrating achievements, and setting intentions for continued well-being.

Holistic Approach to Weight Loss:

- **Mindful Eating Practices:**
  - ◦ The challenge incorporates mindfulness into dietary habits.
  - ◦ Encourage participants to practice mindful eating, fostering awareness of hunger and fullness cues.

- **Stress Reduction for Weight Management:**
  - ◦ Integrate stress-reducing practices within the challenge, such as meditation and deep breathing.
  - ◦ Stress management is vital for weight loss, as it mitigates the impact of stress hormones on the body.

- **Daily Movement for Caloric Expenditure:**
  - ◦ Chair yoga sessions contribute to daily caloric expenditure.
  - ◦ The challenge promotes weight loss through the combination of mindful movement and enhanced physical activity.

- **Enhanced Sleep for Weight Regulation:**
  - ◦ Emphasize the importance of quality sleep for weight regulation.
  - ◦ Chair yoga practices for better sleep are included in the challenge to support overall well-being.

- **Community Engagement and Accountability:**
  - ◦ Foster a sense of community through online

forums or social media.

  ○ Accountability and shared experiences create a supportive environment, enhancing the likelihood of adherence to the challenge.

Physical and Mental Benefits of the 21-Day Chair Yoga Challenge:

- **Weight Loss and Caloric Expenditure:**
  ○ Consistent chair yoga practice contributes to calorie burning, supporting weight loss efforts.
  ○ Dynamic flows and core-strengthening poses enhance metabolism and promote a gradual and sustainable weight loss journey.

- **Improved Flexibility and Mobility:**
  ○ The challenge's focus on flexibility contributes to improved joint health and enhanced overall mobility.
  ○ Increased flexibility aids in achieving a wider range of motion during chair yoga poses.

- **Enhanced Core Strength:**
  ○ Core-strengthening poses target abdominal muscles, promoting a strong and stable core.
  ○ Improved core strength contributes to better posture, balance, and overall physical well-being.

- **Stress Reduction and Mental Well-Being:**
  ○ Daily mindfulness practices within the challenge reduce stress levels.
  ○ Stress reduction supports mental well-being, fostering a positive mindset conducive to sustainable weight loss.

- **Improved Sleep Quality:**
  ○ Chair yoga practices specifically designed for

better sleep contribute to improved sleep quality.

- Enhanced sleep supports overall health and aids in weight management.

- **Increased Energy Levels:**
  - The challenge's energizing flows and sequences contribute to increased energy levels.
  - Participants experience a revitalized sense of well-being, promoting a more active lifestyle.

Practical Tips for Success in the 21-Day Chair Yoga Challenge:

- **Set Realistic Goals:**
  - Encourage participants to set achievable and realistic goals for the challenge.
  - Realistic goals foster a sense of accomplishment and motivation.

- **Listen to the Body:**
  - Emphasize the importance of listening to the body's signals during chair yoga practice.
  - Participants should honor their comfort levels and modify poses as needed.

- **Hydration and Nutrition:**
  - Highlight the significance of staying hydrated and nourishing the body with wholesome foods.
  - Adequate hydration and nutrition complement the benefits of chair yoga.

- **Create a Supportive Environment:**
  - Foster a supportive community through online platforms or local groups.
  - Shared experiences and support create a positive and encouraging environment.

- **Celebrate Milestones:**
    - ◦ Encourage participants to celebrate achievements and milestones throughout the challenge.
    - ◦ Recognizing progress fosters a positive mindset and motivation to continue the journey.
- **Integrate Self-Reflection:**
    - ◦ Incorporate self-reflection practices within the challenge.
    - ◦ Journaling or mindfulness exercises encourage participants to connect with their evolving physical and mental states.

Scientific Insights into Chair Yoga and Weight Loss:

- **Cortisol Regulation:**
    - ◦ Chair yoga's stress-reducing effects contribute to cortisol regulation.
    - ◦ Balanced cortisol levels are associated with weight management and reduced abdominal fat.
- **Mind-Body Connection and Eating Behaviors:**
    - ◦ Mindful practices within chair yoga positively impact eating behaviors.
    - ◦ Mindful eating has been linked to healthier food choices and improved weight management.
- **Increased Physical Activity and Metabolism:**
    - ◦ Chair yoga contributes to increased physical activity levels.
    - ◦ Enhanced physical activity, even in a seated practice, supports metabolism and weight loss.
- **Improved Sleep and Weight Loss:**
    - ◦ Quality sleep is linked to weight regulation.

    ◦ Chair yoga practices for better sleep contribute to improved sleep quality, supporting weight loss efforts.

Conclusion:

In conclusion, the 21-Day Chair Yoga Challenge emerges as a transformative and accessible journey toward weight loss and overall well-being. This comprehensive guide has explored the foundations of the challenge, the daily practices, and the holistic approach to weight loss. By blending the principles of chair yoga, mindful eating, and self-care, participants embark on a 21-day journey that extends beyond physical transformation. The challenge becomes a catalyst for cultivating a positive relationship with the body, embracing mindfulness, and fostering sustainable habits for long-term well-being. As individuals immerse themselves in the 21-Day Chair Yoga Challenge, they unlock the potential for physical vitality, mental clarity, and a profound sense of self-discovery—a journey that extends far beyond the initial 21 days, laying the groundwork for a healthier and more balanced lifestyle.

The End.

www.ingramcontent.com/pod-product-compliance
Lightning Source LLC
Chambersburg PA
CBHW070812260726
48660CB00005B/1822